Pra
OBSTETRICS
and
GYNECOLOGY

Practice Guidelines for OBSTETRICS and GYNECOLOGY

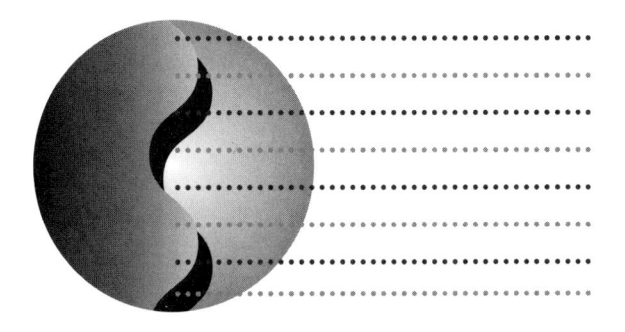

Janet Scoggin, CNM, PhD
Arizona State University
College of Nursing
Associate Clinical Professor
Director of Women's Health Care
    Nurse Practitioner Program
Tempe, Arizona

Geri Morgan, CNM, ND
Women's Healthcare Associates
Director of Provider Services
Certified Nurse-Midwife
Tempe, Arizona

Arizona State University
College of Nursing
Adjunct Faculty
Tempe, Arizona

Lippincott
Philadelphia • New York

Acquisitions Editor: Jennifer E. Brogan
Coordinating Editorial Assistant: Susan V. Barta
Project Editor: Gretchen Metzger
Production Manager: Helen Ewan
Production Coordinator: Kathryn Rule
Design Coordinator: Doug Smock
Indexer: Michael Ferreira

Copyright © 1997 by Lippincott-Raven Publishers. All rights reserved. This book is protected by copyright. No part of it may be reproduced, stored in a retrieval system, or transmitted, in any form or by any means—electronic, mechanical, photocopying, recording, or otherwise—without the prior written permission of the publisher, except for brief quotations embodied in critical articles and reviews and testing and evaluation materials provided by publisher to instructors whose schools have adopted its accompanying textbook. Printed in the United States of America. For information write Lippincott-Raven Publishers, 227 East Washington Square, Philadelphia, PA 19106-3780.

Materials appearing in this book prepared by individuals as part of their official duties as U.S. Government employees are not covered by the above-mentioned copyright.

9 8 7 6 5 4 3 2 1

Library of Congress Cataloging-in-Publication Data
Scoggin, Janet.
  Practice guidelines for obstetrics and gynecology / by Janet
  Scoggin, Geri Morgan.
    p.   cm.
  Includes bibliographical references and index.
  ISBN 0-397-55426-5 (pbk. : alk. paper)
  1. Obstetrics—Outlines, syllabi, etc.   2. Gynecology—Outlines,
syllabi, etc.   3. Women—Health and hygiene—Outlines, syllabi, etc.
I. Morgan, Geri. II. Title.
  [DNLM: 1. Obstetrics—handbooks.   2. Genital Diseases, Female–
–handbooks.   3. Drugs—handbooks.   WQ 39 S422p   1997]
RG101.S3577   1997
618—dc20
DNLM/DLC
for Library of Congress   96-31549
                                                                         CIP

Care has been taken to confirm the accuracy of the information presented and to describe generally accepted practices. However, the authors, editors, and publisher are not responsible for errors or omissions or for any consequences from application of the information in this book and make no warranty, express or implied, with respect to the contents of the publication.

The authors, editors and publisher have exerted every effort to ensure that drug selection and dosage set forth in this text are in accordance with current recommendations and practice at the time of publication. However, in view of ongoing research, changes in government regulations, and the constant flow of information relating to drug therapy and drug reactions, the reader is urged to check the package insert for each drug for any change in indications and dosage and for added warnings and precautions. This is particularly important when the recommended agent is a new or infrequently employed drug.

Some drugs and medical devices presented in this publication have Food and Drug Administration (FDA) clearance for limited use in restricted research settings. It is the responsibility of the health care provider to ascertain the FDA status of each drug or device planned for use in their clinical practice.

DEDICATION

This book is dedicated to all the health professionals that will use it. Our hope is that they will look beyond technology and truly learn to be "with woman:" to listen to her, to respect her choices, and to protect her life and that of her child.

—J.S.

To everyone who has touched my life—without them, this book would not have been possible.

— G.M.

Preface

Several years ago, both of the nurse–midwife authors were working together in a large practice with several obstetricians and nurse practitioners and a physician's assistant. We began to realize the need to have guidelines for practice so that all the practitioners would know what to expect of each other regarding patient management. These practice guidelines were developed as an aid to uniform quality of care and as a quick clinical reference. These guidelines have continued to grow throughout the years even though one of us has since left the practice for an academic position. The author still in the practice has been faithful in updating and adding pertinent information to the guidelines; the academician has used them to teach her women's health care practitioner students clinical thinking and management skills.

We have chosen to design a book of guidelines rather than use the older format of *protocol*. Protocols have become connected with a rigid set of correct procedures, whereas guidelines leave more room for the exercise of clinical judgement in individual circumstances (American College of Nurse–Midwives, 1995). Guidelines provide a system for handling problems and are particularly useful when multiple health personnel are involved. Guidelines allow practitioners to communicate with each other and with their collaborating physicians as to what will usually be done in a specific situation.

This book, which is in outline form, is designed as a quick resource for all who care for the health needs of women: nurse–midwives, nurse practitioners, physician assistants, medical students, residents, and interns. It uses principles and knowledge from the fields of midwifery, nursing, and medicine, applying them to women's health care throughout the life cycle.

Part I is an overview of well woman care in gynecology as well as obstetrics. It outlines basic history-taking and physical examination procedures, as well as lab work and teaching needed in both situations. Included in this section are discussions of screening tests, contraceptive methods, the initial prenatal visit, return prenatal visit, and nutrition and weight gain in pregnancy. For nurse–midwives or other practitioners who will be attending deliveries, guidelines for intrapartum and postpartum care are included.

Part II features common discomforts of pregnancy. These discomforts have been organized alphabetically in a convenient table format for quick reference. The table includes etiology, differential diagnosis, relief measures, and danger signs.

Part III is concerned with the management of common gynecologic and obstetric problems and procedures. Most topics are initiated with a definition of the condition, followed by its etiology, clinical features (including history, signs, and symptoms), and management. The topics in this chapter are listed in alphabetical order for ease of reference.

Part IV is a concise review of the drugs referred to in the book and commonly used in women's health care. The drugs suggested in this book for the treatment of various conditions are recommended in the medical literature and conform to accepted medical practice. Because there is often change in type and dosage of therapeutic regimens, it is recommended that practitioners check updated literature and package inserts for revised recommendations. The drug index includes dosages, pregnancy category classification, side effects, drug interactions, and patient education.

Contents

PART I: GUIDELINES FOR WELL WOMAN CARE 1
Janet Scoggin and Geri Morgan
Gynecologic Care. 3
Contraception 7
Contraceptive Methods 8
Care During Pregnancy 25
Nutrition and Weight Gain in Pregnancy 31
Care During Labor and Delivery 33
Laboratory Studies. 41

PART II: COMMON DISCOMFORTS OF PREGNANCY. 47
Anita Pendo

PART III: MANAGEMENT OF COMMON PROBLEMS AND PROCEDURES 65
Janet Scoggin and Geri Morgan
Abruptio Placenta. 67
Amenorrhea. 69
Anemia. 72
Anemia: Acquired Hemolytic. 75
Anemia: Iron Deficiency 77
Anemia: Megaloblastic. 79
Anemia: Pernicious 80
Anemia: Sickle Cell 81
Backache 82
Bacterial Vaginosis. 83
Bleeding in Pregnancy Under 20 Weeks' Gestation. 85
Bleeding in Pregnancy Over 20 Weeks' Gestation. 89
Breech Presentation. 91
Cardiovascular Assessment 92

Cervical Abnormalities... 94
Chlamydia... 96
Colds, Flu, Upper Respiratory Infection... 99
Coughs... 100
Diabetes Mellitus... 102
Diarrhea... 107
Dysfunctional Uterine Bleeding... 109
Dysmenorrhea... 112
Ectopic Pregnancy... 117
Edema in Pregnancy... 119
Endometrial Biopsy... 121
Endometritis... 123
Establishing the Estimated Date of Confinement (EDC)... 126
Fetal Heart Tones... 128
Fetal Movement... 130
Galactorrhea... 132
Genetic Screening... 133
Gonorrhea... 137
Grand Multiparity... 141
Headache... 142
HELLP Syndrome... 144
Hemorrhoids... 146
Hepatitis... 147
Herpes Simplex... 152
Human Immunodeficiency Viral Disease (HIV)... 157
Human Papilloma Virus/Condylomata Acuminata... 159
Hydatidiform Mole... 161
Hypertension During Pregnancy... 163
Intrauterine Fetal Growth Retardation... 166
Isoimmunization... 168
Lupus... 171
Mammography... 173
Mastitis... 174
Menopause/Perimenopause... 176
Monilia Vaginitis... 182
Multiple Pregnancy... 184
Non-Stress Test... 186
Papanicolaou (Pap) Smear... 187
Pediculosis Pubis... 187
Placenta Previa... 191
Pneumonia... 193
Polyhydramnios... 196
Postmaturity... 198
Postpartum Hemorrhage... 200
Premature Rupture of Membranes... 204

Prematurity.. 207
Pruritus in Pregnancy.. 210
Puerperal Infection... 212
Rashes... 214
Round Ligament Pain.. 221
Rubella... 222
Scabies... 224
Skin Conditions in Pregnancy..................................... 226
Sore Throat... 231
Syphilis... 232
Thrombophlebitis... 236
Thyroid Disease... 238
Trichomonas Vaginitis... 240
Tuberculosis.. 242
Urinary Tract Infections... 244
Vaccinations.. 248
Vaginal Discharge.. 249

PART IV: DRUG INDEX 255
Janet Scoggin and Geri Morgan
Actifed... 258
Acyclovir... 259
Amoxicillin.. 259
Ampicillin... 260
Aspirin... 261
AZT.. 262
Bellergal-S.. 263
Benadryl... 264
Bethamethasone dipropionate.................................. 264
Bicillin Long-Acting.. 265
Cholestyramine... 266
Chromagen... 266
Cleocin/Cleocin Vaginal.. 267
Climara.. 268
Colace... 268
Darvocet N-100... 269
Demerol... 269
Depo-Provera.. 270
Diflucan... 270
Doxycycline.. 271
Emetrol.. 271
Entex/Entex LA... 272
Epinephrine.. 272
Erythromycin, E.E.S., E-mycin................................... 273

Estrace/Estradiol 0.01% Vaginal Cream............................. 274
Estraderm Transdermal Patch 275
Estratest/Estratest H.S... 276
Ethambutol.. 277
Famvir 277
Femstat... 278
Ferrous Sulfate 278
Fioricet... 279
Fiorinal... 279
Flagyl 280
Fleet Enema 280
Floxin.. 281
Folic Acid 281
Fosamax.. 282
Glycerin Suppository 282
Hemabate 283
Hepatitis B Vaccine... 283
Hydroxychloroquine 284
Ibuprofen 284
Immune Globulin (IG).. 285
Isoniazid 286
Keflex.. 286
Macrobid... 287
Macrodantin.. 287
Magnesium Sulfate... 288
Metamucil 288
Methergine... 289
MetroGel-Vaginal.. 289
Micronor... 290
Milk of Magnesia 290
Monistat 7/Monistat 3 291
Nizoral 291
Nonoxynol-9 292
Norplant... 292
Nucofed 293
Nystatin 200,000 Units.. 293
Ogen 0.625 mg Tablets/Ogen Vaginal Cream 294
Phenergan/Phenergan VC 294
Pitocin... 295
Prednisolone.. 296
Prednisone 297
Premarin (Oral/Cream) 298
Premphase 299
Prempro 300
Preparation H 300

Probenecid 301
Proctofoam-HC. 301
Progesterone in Oil. 302
Promethazine HCL 302
Prostin E2, Prepidil Gel. 303
Proventil Inhaler. 303
Provera 304
Pyrazinamide 305
RhoGAM 305
Rifampin. 306
Rocephin 306
Rubella Virus Vaccine. 307
Senokot 307
Slow Fe/Slow Fe Plus Folic Acid 308
Spectinomycin 308
Stadol 309
Sudafed/Sudafed 12 Hour Capsules 309
Terazol 3/Terazol 7/Terazol Cream 310
Terbutaline 310
Tetracycline 311
Tigan. 311
Tums. 312
Tylenol 312
Tylenol #3. 313
Unisom 313
Vistaril, Atarax, Anxanil. 314
Zantac. 314
Zidovudine 315
Zithromax. 315
Bibliography **317**
Appendix **321**
Index **327**

I

Guidelines for Well Woman Care

GYNECOLOGIC CARE

For many women, visits to gynecologic care providers are their sole source of preventive health care. Therefore, these visits must be comprehensive and accomplish the following three purposes: (1) detection, diagnosis, and treatment of gynecologic problems; (2) screening for other health problems; and (3) general health maintenance and prevention of illness.[1] To accomplish these purposes, the practitioner must take a detailed history and perform a thorough physical exam. The proper understanding and use of screening tests is also necessary.

I. **History Taking**
   A. Identification information
   B. Reason for visit: Why has the woman sought care?
   C. Menstrual history: First day and duration of the last menstrual period; age at menarche; usual interval, duration, and amount of menses; spotting or cramps midcycle; any significant problems such as cramping, nausea, depression, and so on.
   D. Gynecologic history: Past and current gynecologic problems, genitourinary disorders, vaginitis, sexually transmitted diseases (STDs), infertility.
   E. Obstetric (OB) history: Gravidy (number of pregnancies), parity (number of viable pregnancies), course of pregnancies and labor, problems with pregnancies, labor, deliveries, postpartum.
   F. Contraceptive history: Types and satisfaction with current and previously used contraceptives.
   G. Medical history: Complete medical history including substance use, allergies, any previous transfusions, and exposure to diethylstilbestrol.
   H. Surgical history: Circumstances of any previous surgeries.
   I. Family history: Chronic diseases of first-degree family members: diabetes, cancer, cardiac disease, osteoporosis.
   J. Social/cultural history: Support system, cultural background, living situation.
   K. Occupational history: Possible exposure to toxic substances, heavy lifting, standing or sitting too long, night work.
   L. Sexual history: Sexually active? Sexual preference, number of partners, any problems with intercourse.
   M. Nutritional history: 24-hour diet recall, caffeine, usual weight, recent weight changes, eating disorders.
   N. Activity/exercise history: Activities of daily living, regular exercise?

II. **Physical Exam**
   A. General: Height, weight, blood pressure, pulse, temperature.
   B. Head and neck: Inspect eyes, ears, nose, mouth, oropharynx, tongue, thyroid gland.

---
[1] Lichtman R, Papera S. 1990.

C. Lymph nodes: Palpate and inspect anterior and posterior cervical, submental, supraclavicular, axillary, epitrochlear, and inguinal.
D. Back: Inspect straightness, palpate for costovertebral angle tenderness.
E. Lungs: Inspect, percuss, auscultate.
F. Heart: Auscultate for rate, rhythm, regularity, murmurs, extra heart sounds.
G. Breasts
   1. Inspect in three positions: arms at side, over the head, and pressed against hips with elbows extended laterally. Look for symmetry, nipple alignment, abnormal venous pattern, coloration and skin appearance, and changes including dimpling and puckering.
   2. Palpate all four quadrants of each breast with patient lying down and arm over her head on the side being examined. Use radial or transverse techniques. Note size, shape, consistency, tenderness, and nodularity.
   3. Inspect nipples for eversion, note any discharge following expression.
   4. Palpate subclavicular area noting masses or tenderness.
H. Abdomen: Inspect for contour, scars, masses. Palpate for masses, liver, spleen, or kidney enlargement and tenderness.
I. Lower extremities: Inspect and palpate noting varicosities, lesions, edema, erythema, warmth, and pain.
J. Pelvis
   1. Inspect external genitalia for lesions, scars, configurations.
   2. Palpate Bartholin's and Skene's glands, note urethral discharge.
   3. Perform speculum exam to observe vagina and cervix.
      a. Note color of the cervix, any erythema, irregularities, lesions, ectropion or friability, configuration of the os, discharge. Obtain Papanicolaou (Pap) smear and any necessary cultures.
      b. Inspect the vagina. Note the color, rugation, and presence of any abnormality or discharge.
   4. Perform bimanual exam to evaluate uterus and adnexa, noting contour, nodularity, position, size, and tenderness.
   5. Perform rectal exam if indicated.

III. **Recommendations for Preventive and Screening Tests for Women:** Clinicians often see women whose medical problems could have been avoided with proper prevention and screening. Despite the benefits, preventive services should be used selectively. One should be confident that the tests' ability to detect disease will be greater than any harm done or excessive cost.

The efficacy of the preventive and screening tests shown in Table 1-1 have been thoroughly evaluated by the Canadian Task Force (CTF) (1987), the United States Preventive Services Task Force (USPSTF), the American College of Physicians (ACP)[2] and the American College of Ob-

(text continues on page 7)

---
[2]Eddy DM. 1991.

Table 1-1. Prevention and Screening Recommendations for Women*

Intervention	Health Condition	Target Group	Recommendations
Blood Pressure	CHD, cerebrovascular disease, renal disease		
Routine		18 yr+	Every 1–2 yr
High risk		18 yr+, diastolic BP is 85–90 mmHg, 1 or more CHD risk factors present	Every yr
Clinician Breast Examination	Breast cancer		
Routine		18 yr+ (ACOG)	Every yr
High risk		18 yr+ (ACP), 35 yr+ (CTF, USPTSTF), history of premenopausal breast cancer in a first-degree family member.	Every yr
Mammography	Breast cancer		
Routine		50–75 yr+	Every yr (ACP, CTF, ACOG)
		40–50 yr	Every 1–2 yr (USPSTF, ACOG)
High risk		30–40 yr, history of premenopausal breast cancer in a first-degree family member, other risk factors (ACP)	Every yr (ACP, CTF, USPSTF)
Papanicolaou Smear	Cervical cancer		
Routine		18 yr+, no other risk factors	Every 1–3 yr
High risk		18 yr+ or onset of intercourse, presence of risk factors	Every yr

(*continued*)

Table 1-1. (Continued)

Intervention	Health Condition	Target Group	Recommendations
Sigmoidoscopy	Colorectal cancer		
Routine		50 yr+ (ACP)	Every 3–5 yr (ACP)
High risk		40 yr+ (CTF), 50 yr+ (USPSTF), hx one first-degree family member with colon cancer or personal hx of endometrial, ovarian, or breast cancer	Every 3–5 yr (CTF, USPSTF)
Colonoscopy	Colorectal cancer		
Very high risk		More than 1 first-degree family member with colon cancer (especially if <40 yr at diagnosis); familial polyposis coli; personal hx colon cancer, ulcerative colitis, 10 yr of adenomatous polyps	Every 3–5 yr (ACP, CTF, USPSTF)
Hemocult	Colorectal cancer	40+ yr (ACOG)	Every yr
Nonfasting Cholesterol	CHD		
Routine		18 yr+ (ACP, USPSTF)	Every 5 yr
High risk		18 yr+, 1 or more CHD risk factors	More frequently (ACP, USPSTF) individual clinical judgment (CTF)

ACOG = American College of Obstetricians & Gynecologists; ACP = American College of Physicians; CHD = congenital heart disease; CTF = Canadian Task Force; and USPSTF = United States Preventive Services Task Force.
*Adapted from Lemcke DP, Pattison J, Marshall LA, Cowley DS. 1995; 51–52.

stetricians & Gynecologists (ACOG). The emphasis is on services for which the evidence of prevention are the strongest.

CONTRACEPTION

I. **Contraception Should Be Discussed with Patients**
   A. At the annual exam
   B. When the patient comes to the office for a pregnancy test
   C. During the last trimester of pregnancy
   D. During the first few days postpartum
   E. At the postpartum office visit, usually at 6 weeks
   F. At any other time the patient requests it

II. **Method Desired:** Unless the patient is absolutely sure which contraceptive method she desires (or if she desires not to use contraception), the following should be done:
   A. Contraceptive history
      1. What methods has the patient used in the past?
      2. How long did she use each method?
      3. Any complications from any method?
      4. What was her level of satisfaction with each method?
      5. Why did she discontinue using each method?
      6. Would she consider using a method she has used in the past? Why or why not?
   B. Health history
   C. Physical exam if not done within the past year
   D. Labwork
      1. Pap smear
      2. Hematocrit
      3. GC and chlamydia screening if indicated
   E. Counseling: Offer information about methods the patient has not used, and/or give handout comparing methods. Find out how much she knows about each method, whether she has misinformation, and if she is interested in any particular method. If the patient desires, help her explore which contraceptive method would be best for her. May use the questionnaire in *Contraceptive Technology*, "Am I Going to Like This Method of Birth Control?"[3] Factors that may influence her selection include:
      1. Social/cultural trends
         a. Interest in a method that is currently popular
         b. Family background

---
[3]Hatcher RA, Stewart F, Trussell J. 1990.

     c. Lifestyle
     d. Partner cooperativeness with contraception
  2. Religion
     Prohibition of some, or all, methods
  3. Psychological factors
     a. Negative or positive feelings about certain methods
     b. Recent negative publicity about a certain method
     c. Unfavorable past experience with a certain method
  4. Technicalities
     a. Ease of use may or may not be an important consideration for the patient
     b. Ability to master the technique involved in using certain methods
     c. Access to medical care
  5. Frequency of sexual intercourse, number of partners
     a. If infrequent, a barrier method may be preferable to the upkeep and potential complications of other methods.
     b. If multiple partners, at more risk for STDs and pelvic inflammatory disease (PID), intrauterine device (IUD) would not be ideal choice but barrier methods may provide some protection.
  6. Ability to comply with the requirements of a contraceptive method. Examine whether patient is likely to use a coitus-related method or remember to take a pill every day.
  7. Length of anticipated use of a contraceptive method. If needed for only a few months until husband gets vasectomy, the birth control pill (BCP) is not worth the effort or potential side effects.
  8. Possible side effects and questions of safety related to the method:
     a. The patient must decide what risks she is willing to take.
     b. Both positive and negative side effects should be discussed.
  9. Effectiveness of a contraceptive method. High priority if a subsequent pregnancy would be unacceptable and/or if abortion is not an option.
  10. Cost of contraceptive method: Will her insurance company pay for this method?
  11. Reversibility of a contraceptive method
      a. IUDs may impair fertility
      b. Sterilization can sometimes be reversed with surgery but should be considered permanent.

CONTRACEPTIVE METHODS

I. Cervical Cap
   A. Definition: The cervical cap is a barrier method of contraception, similar to the diaphragm, except that it fits over just the cervix to prevent sperm from entering the uterus.

B. Effectiveness: The effectiveness rate is between 82% and 90%. Effectiveness increases with the length of time a person has used this method. Older women report a higher success rate.

C. Advantages
  1. It can be left in place up to 24 to 36 hours.
  2. It does not require a spermicide.

D. Disadvantages
  1. There are only four sizes, making it difficult to fit.
  2. Because of cervical position, size, and so on, only 50% of women can be fitted.
  3. After 12 to 24 hours in place, there may be an increased incidence of foul-smelling discharge.
  4. Manual dexterity is needed to properly place the cervical cap.
  5. It should not be used on heavy flow days of the menstrual period because this may cause menstrual regurgitation into the Fallopian tubes and predispose to endometriosis. Should be removed 6 to 8 hours after intercourse on lighter flow days.
  6. Has been implicated in cervical ulcers, spread of human papilloma virus
  7. May provide less protection from STDs than a diaphragm.

E. Management
  1. After the patient is fitted, she needs to demonstrate an ability to insert, check for correct position, and remove the cap.
  2. Patients who have had an abnormal Pap or history of human papilloma virus on the cervix with treatment by cryosurgery, laser, or loop electrosurgical excision procedure (LEEP) are not good candidates for the cervical cap.

F. Teaching
  1. Proper care of the cap is the same as for the diaphragm.
  2. Pregnancy or a weight loss or gain over 30 pounds may change the cervix. Refitting may be necessary.

II. Condom

A. Definition: A rubber sheath worn over the penis in coitus to prevent impregnation or infection.
  1. Ninety-nine percent of condoms are made of latex, which provides protection against pregnancy because sperm cannot penetrate the condom. Other organisms that cause STDs, human papilloma virus, and human immunodeficiency virus (HIV), do not penetrate latex condoms but may penetrate condoms made from intestine (eg, "Natural Skin").
  2. Some condoms come with spermicide, which increases the effectiveness.

B. Effectiveness: 85% to 89%
  1. Inconsistent use accounts for most failures.
  2. Breakage has been reported from as low as 1 to as high as 12 per 100 episodes of vaginal intercourse.

3. Because leakage of sperm may occur with arousal, the condom must be worn before sexual contact.
C. Advantages
 1. Provides significant protection against STDs.
 2. Cheap
 3. Easy access—condoms are sold over the counter.
D. Disadvantages
 1. There are more effective methods to prevent pregnancy.
 2. Must be applied to penis just before intercourse.
 3. Up to 5% of the population have an allergic response to either the latex or the spermicide.
E. Management
 1. Must be used every time before sexual intercourse.
 2. Use with spermicide is recommended because effectiveness is increased by 5% to 7%.
 3. Directions for each individual spermicide need to be read and followed exactly concerning time of insertion, length of effectiveness, and so on.

III. Depo-Provera Contraceptive Injection

A. Definition: A medroxy progesterone acetate suspension.
B. Effectiveness: Less than 1% of patients using Depo-Provera will become pregnant provided they receive their injection every 12 weeks.
C. Advantages
 1. Does not contain estrogen
 2. One injection of 150 mg intramuscularly (IM) will give protection for 12 weeks.
 3. Convenient
 4. Reversible: 66% of former Depo-Provera users can be expected to become pregnant within 1 year of their last injection. 93% will be pregnant within 24 months.
 5. Can be used by nursing mothers
D. Disadvantages
 1. Irregular or unpredictable bleeding
   a. Bleeding is usually less over time, but irregular.
   b. Amenorrhea may result in 60% to 80% of users by 1 year.
   c. 0.5% of users will experience heavy bleeding.
 2. May decrease calcium and minerals stored in bones.
 3. Other side effects
   a. Increased appetite (may increase weight)
   b. Headaches
   c. Temporary hair loss
   d. Stomach cramps: Often noted within the first 2 weeks of the injection and tend to decrease until the next injection.

  e. Fatigue
  f. Decreased sex drive
 4. Does not protect against STDs
E. Contraindications
 1. Pregnancy
 2. Allergy to Depo-Provera
 3. Current liver disease
 4. Undiagnosed uterine bleeding
F. Management
 1. Use
  a. 150 mg IM every 12 weeks +/− 1 to 2 weeks
  b. The medication should be started within 5 days of a menstrual cycle or within 4 weeks of delivery if not breastfeeding, and by 6 weeks after delivery if breastfeeding to ensure against pregnancy.
  c. If the patient has amenorrhea or it has been over 14 weeks since her last injection, a pregnancy test needs to be done before her next injection.
 2. Side effects
  a. Breakthrough bleeding may sometimes be controlled by giving 1 to 2 cycles of a low-dose BCP.
  b. Post Depo-Provera amenorrhea
   (1) Before 5 months, reassure patient that it sometimes takes awhile for her periods to restart.
   (2) After 5 months, the patient may be cycled with estrogen/progesterone (BCPs), after pregnancy has been ruled out. If she does not have withdrawal bleeding after the second cycle, adding 1 to 2 mg of estradiol (Estrace) or other estrogen to the first 3 weeks of the BCP may prime the endometrium.

IV. Diaphragm
 A. Definition: A small rubber cup with a rim stabilized by a rubber-covered steel spring. It fits in the vaginal vault, forming a barrier between the sperm and the cervix. It is used with spermicidal jelly or cream to increase effectiveness.
 B. Effectiveness
  1. Theoretical: 97%
  2. Use: 85%
 C. Advantages
  1. Minimal side effects
  2. Protective of STDs
 D. Disadvantages
  1. Discomfort from poorly fitted diaphragm
  2. Perceived interference with spontaneity of lovemaking
  3. Perceived messiness
  4. Can cause bladder infections

E. Contraindications
  1. Absolute
     a. Allergy to rubber, spermicide, or both
     b. Inability of patient or partner to learn correct insertion technique
     c. Recurrent urinary tract infections (UTIs)
     d. Inability to achieve satisfactory fitting
     e. History of toxic shock syndrome
     f. Severe uterine prolapse, anteversion, or retroversion
     g. Severe cystocele
     h. Rectal or vaginal fistulas
  2. Temporary
     a. Postpartum involution incomplete: Wait at least 6 weeks after delivery before fitting and longer if involution did not occur normally.
     b. Pelvic infection or surgery (eg, PID, spontaneous): Wait until condition resolves, usually about 1 month.
F. Management
  1. Fitting the diaphragm
     a. The patient should be a candidate for a diaphragm as determined by the above screening process.
     b. Selection of type of diaphragm most appropriate
        (1) Flat spring (Ortho)
           (a) Must have strong vaginal support
           (b) Useful for a shallow arch behind the symphysis pubis
        (2) Coil spring (Ortho)
           (a) Average vaginal support is adequate
           (b) Useful for a deep arch behind the symphysis pubis
        (3) Arcing spring (Ortho)
           (a) Provides the most support, therefore, is useful for a patient with less than adequate vaginal or uterine support, that is, almost any woman who has had a vaginal delivery.
           (b) May use it for all women except those with exceptionally firm vaginal tone and those who find the arcing spring uncomfortable.
        (4) Wide seal arching (Milex)
           (a) Is useful for most patients
           (b) Claims to make a more effective seal
     c. The patient should be fitted for the diaphragm according to technique outlined in textbooks.
     d. If this is the first time the patient has used a diaphragm, have her practice inserting it, checking for proper placement, and removing it at the office visit.

e. Give the patient printed instructions, which include:
     (1) How to insert, remove, and care for the diaphragm.
     (2) How to use the diaphragm.
     (3) How to avoid toxic shock syndrome:
        (a) Do not wear the diaphragm during menses.
        (b) Avoid leaving the diaphragm in place longer than 24 hours.
        (c) If the following danger signs appear, call the health care provider, or seek other medical help immediately.
           i. Fever (temperature of 101°F or more)
           ii. Diarrhea
           iii. Vomiting
           iv. Muscle aches
           v. Sunburn-like rash

2. Follow-up: If this is the first time the patient has used a diaphragm, instruct her to return in 2 to 4 weeks with the diaphragm in place. At this visit, the following history and physical should be done.
   a. History
      (1) How many times was the diaphragm worn?
      (2) What is the longest period of time it was left in place?
      (3) Were there any signs that the diaphragm is too large?
         (a) Pain in the abdomen, back, or rectum
         (b) Thigh cramps
         (c) Difficulty voiding
      (4) Any difficulty with
         (a) Preparation for insertion
         (b) Insertion of diaphragm
         (c) Checking for proper alignment
         (d) Removal of diaphragm
      (5) Are she and her partner satisfied with the method?
   b. Pelvic exam
      (1) Check for proper placement of the diaphragm.
      (2) Check for fit and continuing correctness of type and size.
      (3) Check for pelvic pain and vaginal irritation.
   c. Instruct the patient to return if at any time she has difficulty with the diaphragm and/or
      (1) She experiences any discomfort with the diaphragm.
      (2) Her diaphragm is damaged or deteriorating
      (3) Her diaphragm needs to be refitted:
         (a) After having a baby.
         (b) After any pelvic surgery.
         (c) If she gains or loses 20 pounds or more.

(d) If the diaphragm was initially fitted before the patient had experienced at least 20 acts of coitus.

(4) She desires a different method of contraception

V. Intrauterine Device

  A. Definition: A contraceptive device made of plastic with or without copper or Progestasert.

    It is introduced into the endometrial cavity through the cervical canal and has a monofilament nylon tail that protrudes from the cervix into the vagina. It acts to prevent conception by immobilization of sperm, increased motility of ovum through the Fallopian tube, and establishing an inflammatory response, causing lysis of sperm and the blastocyst.

  B. Effectiveness
1. 94% effective the first year
2. 96% effective the next 9 years

  C. Advantages
1. Relatively carefree method
2. Highly effective

  D. Disadvantages
1. Heavier menstrual bleeding and/or intramenstrual spotting
2. Pain and cramping (decreases with time)
3. Possible expulsion
4. Possible embedding or perforation of uterus
5. Increased risk of PID

  E. Contraindications
1. Absolute
   a. Nulliparous
   b. Active pelvic infection (acute or subacute), including known or suspected gonorrhea or chlamydia
   c. Known or suspected pregnancy
2. Strong relative
   a. Multiple sexual partners or strong likelihood that the woman will have multiple partners during the time that IUD is in place
   b. Multiple sexual partners by partner of IUD user
   c. Postpartum endometritis or infected abortion within the year
   d. Acute or purulent cervicitis
   e. Bleeding disorders not yet definitively diagnosed
   f. History of ectopic pregnancy or conditions that predispose a woman to it
   g. Single episode of pelvic infection if patient desires subsequent pregnancy
   h. Immunosuppressed—acquired immunodeficiency syndrome, diabetes, corticosteroid treatment, and so forth
   i. Blood coagulation disorders
   j. Previous pregnancy while using the IUD

3. Other conditions that may contraindicate IUD insertion
   a. Valvular heart disease (potentially making patient susceptible to subacute bacterial endocarditis)
   b. Endometrial or cervical malignancy
   c. Severe cervical stenosis
   d. Small uterus that sounds to below 6 cm
   e. Endometriosis
   f. Leiomyomata
   g. Endometrial polyps
   h. Congenital uterine abnormalities or fibroids that prevent proper placement
   i. Severe dysmenorrhea
   j. Heavy menstrual flow, irregular menses, or spotting
   k. Allergy to copper
   l. Anemia
   m. Impaired ability to check for danger signals
   n. Inability to check for IUD string
   o. Past history of gonorrhea, chlamydia, herpes, or syphilis
   p. Genital actinomycosis
   q. Past history of severe vasovagal reactivity or fainting
   r. Previous problems with IUD expulsion
   s. Vaginal discharge or infection
   t. History of pelvic infection
   u. Previous pelvic surgery

F. Management
   1. A complete history and physical, including recent Pap smear, should be on the chart.
      a. If there is a possibility of STDs or pregnancy, these should be ruled out.
      b. Patients who have never been seen need an initial visit, a Pap smear if one was not performed within 1 year, and chlamydia culture. IUD placement will be at the second visit.
   2. All patients must have read, discussed, and signed the IUD consent form.
   3. Timing of IUD insertion
      a. Insertion at any time of the menstrual cycle is acceptable
      b. The infection rate and the expulsion rate are higher when inserted with the menses.
      c. The cervix is equally as dilated at midcycle, therefore, the IUD can be inserted more easily.
      d. Insertion after day 18 of the cycle may result in more pain and bleeding in the short term.
      e. If the patient has had unprotected sex since her last menses and/or delivery, pregnancy should be ruled out.

4. IUD insertion procedure
   a. Move slowly and gently during all phases of IUD insertion. **Always read the manufacturer's instructions for the specific IUD you are inserting.**
   b. One-half hour before the procedure consider giving:
      (1) An antibiotic as a prophylactic against infection.
      (2) Prostaglandin inhibitor, such as ibuprofen for discomfort.
   c. Explain the procedure to help patient relax.
   d. Show and describe the IUD.
   e. Perform a bimanual exam to ascertain the position of the uterus. Perforations occur most often in a retroflexed uterus that was not diagnosed before the IUD was inserted.
   f. View the cervix and wash the cervix with an antiseptic solution, such as a 1:2500 solution of iodine. If iodine is present in the antiseptic solution, rule out an allergy to iodine.
   g. Intracervical local anesthesia may be injected at this point in the insertion process (injected where the tenaculum is to be placed and paracervically).
   h. Grasp the anterior lip of the cervix with a tenaculum about 1.5 to 2.0 cm from the os. Close the single-tooth tenaculum slowly, one notch at a time. (Use of a tenaculum is not always necessary, although it is generally recommended.)
   i. Sound the uterus slowly and gently. Place a cotton swab at the cervix when the sound is all the way in. Remove sound and swab at the same time. This step permits measurement of the depth of the fundus to within 0.25 cm.
   j. Load the IUD into the inserter barrel under sterile conditions.
   k. Apply steady gentle traction on the tenaculum and introduce the inserter barrel through the cervical canal into the fundus.
   l. Insert the IUD into the cavity of the uterus by either plunging the inner plunger into the outer barrel (push technique) or by retracting the outer barrel over the plunger (withdrawal technique). The withdrawal technique is slightly preferred.
   m. If using a tailed IUD, clip the string. Leave about 5 cm (or longer if the patient is immediately postabortal). It is always possible to trim the string at a later date.
   n. Have the patient feel for the string of the IUD before leaving the examining room. She should be instructed to feel for the IUD string after each menses.
   o. Exercise caution when inserting IUDs in parous women who have not been pregnant for several years. They are more likely to experience vasovagal attacks and postinsertion pain, necessitating immediate removal of the IUD. These problems are also more common in women who are anxious or who have a narrow cervical canal, a small uterine cavity, an empty stomach, or a past history of syncopal attacks.
5. A follow-up visit after the first menses is recommended.

G. Side effects and complications
  1. Spotting, bleeding, hemorrhage, and anemia: Approximately 15% of women will have their IUDs removed because of increased menstrual flow, menstrual cramping, spotting, or bleeding.
  2. Cramping and pain
     a. Mild to moderate cramping immediately after insertion and for a few days can be controlled with medication.
     b. Severe cramping
        (1) After insertion may need to remove
        (2) Rule out PID
  3. IUD expulsion, partial or complete
     a. Signs and symptoms—lengthening or no IUD string, increased cramps, intermenstrual and/or postcoital spotting, dyspareunia, increased vaginal discharge
        (1) A partially expelled IUD must be removed.
        (2) A lost IUD string may indicate expulsion, one that has been pulled into the cervical canal or uterus, or a sign of uterine perforation. The cervical canal can be explored for the string. **Never** explore the uterus before ruling out pregnancy.
           (a) An ultrasound or radiograph will show placement.
           (b) When the IUD is in the uterus, the endometrial cavity may be probed with alligator forceps, uterine packing forceps, or a Novak curette.
  4. Uterine perforations: confirm and consult
  5. Pregnancy
     a. There is a higher incidence of spontaneous abortion, septic abortion, and ectopic pregnancy with an IUD in place.
     b. Confirm pregnancy and consult
  6. PID
     a. Remove the IUD as soon as diagnosed.
     b. Treat aggressively
        (1) Cefoxitin 2 g IM plus probenecid, 1 g orally concurrently, or ceftiaxone 250 mg IM, or equivalent cephalosporin plus
        (2) Doxycycline 100 mg orally twice a day for 10 to 14 days

H. Removal
  1. Removals during menses are somewhat easier.
  2. Procedure
     a. Avoid breaking the string by applying gentle, steady traction and removing the IUD slowly. If the IUD does not come out easily, sound the uterus and then slowly rotate the sound 90 degrees.
     b. If gentle traction does not now lead to IUD removal, dilate the cervix with dilators. A paracervical block may be performed before cervical dilation to diminish pain. The cervix may occasionally need to be dilated with a laminaria.

c. Use of a tenaculum to steady the cervix and straighten the anteversion or retroversion may facilitate IUD removal.
  4. Difficulties
     a. If unable to remove, it may be imbedded. Consult for dilatation and curettage.
     b. If no string is seen, see previous information in Side Effects and Complications on p. 17
  5. Pregnancy: If pregnancy occurs with an IUD in place, it is recommended that the IUD be removed.[4]
     a. The abortion rate is 50% to 55% with the device left in, 25% when removed promptly.
     b. Preterm delivery is 20% with the IUD in place, 5% when removed early.
     c. If IUD is left in, sepsis is of serious concern, not only for the fetus but also may result in maternal morbidity and mortality.

VI. Natural Family Planning

A. Definition: A method based on the concept of fertility awareness: the woman's ability to identify certain physiologic changes that occur during her menstrual cycle that indicate fertile and infertile phases. Abstinence is recommended for the fertile period if pregnancy is not desired.

B. Effectiveness
  1. When used to prevent pregnancy, varies from 60% to 90%.
  2. When used to become pregnant, has not been reported.

C. Advantages
  1. Natural method
  2. Promotes communication between couple
  3. Can be used if pregnancy is desired
  4. Can easily be combined with other methods

D. Disadvantages
  1. Relatively high failure rate unless used correctly and consistently
  2. Requires good record keeping
  3. Requires abstinence during the woman's fertile period
  4. Does not work well when menstrual cycles are over 40 days, below 20 days, irregular, or changed by stress, illness, travel, and so on

E. Contraindications: If pregnancy should be avoided due to mental or physical problems, another more effective method needs to be considered.

F. Methods
  1. Basal body temperature (BBT)
     a. BBT is the temperature of the body at complete rest.

---

[4]Cunningham FG, MacDonald P, Grant N. 1989.

b. The BBT method is based on the following facts.
   (1) Estrogen and progesterone, while present throughout the menstrual cycle, rise sharply after ovulation.
   (2) Progesterone causes the BBT to rise several tenths of one degree over what it was before ovulation. This may be a sharp rise in 1 day or a stair-step rise over 2 to 3 days.
   (3) If pregnancy is not desired, safe days begin 4 days after ovulation.
c. To calculate the safe and fertile days
   (1) The temperature needs to be taken every day before rising
   (2) Ovulation has occurred when the recorded temperatures are 0.3 degrees higher for 3 consecutive days than the temperatures recorded for the 6 days before the rise.
d. Teaching
   (1) To avoid pregnancy, do not have intercourse until the fourth day after ovulation.
   (2) It's easier to determine when ovulation has occurred than to know when it will occur. It, therefore, is safer to have sex only after ovulation has occurred.
   (3) This method is more effective when combined with the cervical mucous method.
   (4) If pregnancy is desired, intercourse should occur before and at the time of ovulation.

2. Cervical mucous
   a. The cervical mucous method is based on the following facts.
      (1) Mucous produced by the cervical cells changes during the menstrual cycle.
      (2) After the period, when estrogen is low, mucous is scant. If present, it is sticky and opaque with cellular matter.
      (3) As estrogen levels increase, the mucous increases in amount. It becomes thinner and milkier.
      (4) Just before ovulation, estrogen peaks. The mucous is high in volume and clear. High elasticity is demonstrated by being able to stretch an unbroken thread between fingers. This is called spinnbarkeit. The mucous forms a fern-like pattern when dried on a slide.
      (5) As progesterone rises, the mucous volume decreases. It becomes thick, cloudy white to white yellow with a large amount of cellular matter. This infertile mucous acts as a barrier to sperm ascending the cervical canal.
   b. Teaching
      (1) To be absolutely safe, it is best to abstain from intercourse until after ovulation, when infertile mucous is present.
      (2) Intercourse during menses and after until the presence of any mucous is probably safe.
      (3) This method is more effective when combined with the BBT method.

3. Rhythm: Used alone is unreliable and not recommended
   a. Rhythm method is based on the following facts.
      (1) The egg once released from the ovary will live 12 to 24 hours.
      (2) Sperm may remain alive in the uterus and Fallopian tubes for 72 hours.
      (3) The time before ovulation may vary considerably. The time after ovulation is more consistent at 14 days plus or minus 2 days before menses begins.
   b. To optimize the chance of pregnancy, coitus should occur every day for several days before ovulation. This allows sperm to be in the Fallopian tube when ovulation occurs.
4. Ovulation kits
   a. Expensive but have the advantage of letting the patient know ovulation has occurred
   b. If pregnancy is not desired, intercourse may begin on day 4 after ovulation.

VII. Norplant
A. Definition: Subdermal implants of six nonbiodegradable Silastic rods that release levonorgestrel gradually over 4 to 5 years.
B. Effectiveness
   1. Approximately 99% effective the first year of use.
   2. In the fifth year of use, 96% to 97.5% effective
C. Advantages
   1. Contain progestin only, therefore, without estrogen side effects
   2. Low effective dose causes few alterations in carbohydrate metabolism, blood coagulation factors, blood pressure, or body weight.
   3. Can be used for breastfeeding postpartum women
D. Disadvantages
   1. Irregular bleeding: Occurs in 60% to 80% of patients the first 1 to 3 months after insertion. With continued use, this decreases to 12% to 17% after the first year. BCPs, preferably with levonorgestrel, can be used for 2 to 3 months to help with adjustment.
   2. Depression/mood swings
   3. Weight gain: Progestin does not cause weight gain directly. It has been implicated in increasing appetite. Diet counseling may be of help.
   4. Hair loss: Progestin changes the cycle of hair growth. Time will resolve this problem.
   5. Amenorrhea: Normally occurs in a small percentage of users, pregnancy needs to be ruled out.
   6. Scarring: A small scar may be left at insertion/removal site.
E. Contraindications
   1. Pregnancy
   2. Desire to be pregnant within 1 to 2 years
   3. Undiagnosed abnormal uterine bleeding

F. Complications
   1. Infection at the site: Treat with antibiotics.
   2. Pregnancy: Should pregnancy occur, the Norplant needs to be removed. There are no known fetal problems caused by progestins.
G. Management
   1. Insertion
      a. The patient needs good counseling.
         (1) If pregnancy is desired within 3 to 5 years, another method may be a better choice.
         (2) Irregular bleeding is a common problem. Sixty to seventy percent of Norplants are removed for this problem.
      b. The patient should be having her period or have a negative pregnancy test.
      c. The Norplant kit contains everything needed except lidocaine to be used for local anesthesia.
      d. Follow Norplant directions for insertion.
      e. Counseling after insertion
         (1) Keep dry for 24 hours.
         (2) Loosen gauze if it is too tight.
         (3) Watch for signs/symptoms of infection.
         (4) The arm over implants may be sensitive for 1 to 2 months.
   2. Norplant removal
      a. If pregnancy is not desired, counsel regarding alternate family planning methods.
         (1) The patient may be started on BCPs or an IUD before removal.
         (2) Depo-Provera 150 mg IM may be given the day of removal.
      b. Refer to Norplant directions for removal.
      c. After removal
         (1) Keep arm dry for 24 hours.
         (2) Watch for signs/symptoms of infection.
         (3) Have the patient return in 5 to 7 days to check operation site for infection, healing.

VIII. **Oral Contraceptives**
   A. Definition: Synthetic steroids similar to the estrogens and progestins that are natural female sex hormones. These steroids are used in doses and in combinations that provide contraception by inhibiting ovulation, implantation, or both.
   B. Effectiveness
      1. Theoretical: 99.5% to 100%
      2. Use: 90% to 96%, probably due to errors in usage
   C. Advantages
      1. Menstrual benefits
         a. Less dysmenorrhea and premenstrual tension

b. Lighter periods, resulting in less anemia
   c. Regularity of menstrual periods
  2. Totally self-reliant, does not require partner cooperation
  3. Not coitus-related, allows for spontaneity
  4. Affords protection from the following illnesses:
     a. Decreased risk of PID after being on the pill for 1 year
     b. Decreased risk of endometrial and ovarian cancer
     c. Decreased incidence of ovarian cysts
     d. Decreased incidence of fibroadenomas of the breast and fibrocystic breast disease
D. Disadvantages
  1. Increased risk of
     a. Cardiovascular disease
     b. Liver tumors
     c. Hypertension
  2. Must remember to take the pill daily
  3. Hormonal side effects in some women
E. Contraindications
  1. Absolute
     a. Known or suspected carcinoma of the breast
     b. Known or suspected estrogen-dependent neoplasia
     c. Thromboembolic disease or thrombophlebitis, cerebral vascular disease, coronary artery disease, or history of these conditions
     d. Undiagnosed uterine bleeding
     e. Known or suspected pregnancy
     f. Impaired liver function or hepatic disease
  2. Relative
     a. Hypertension
     b. Migraine headaches
     c. Diabetes or pre-diabetes
     d. Epilepsy or convulsions
     e. Active gallbladder disease
     f. Active phase mononucleosis
     g. Sickle cell trait or disease
     h. Age 45 or older
     i. Ages 35 to 40 and heavy smoker
     j. Lactation: decreases milk supply
F. Management
  1. Initiating the pill
     a. The patient should be a candidate for BCP, as determined by history and physical exam.
     b. Selection of pill most appropriate for individual patient

- (1) In general, prescribe BCP with
  - (a) 35 µg estrogen or less
  - (b) A low-potency progestin
- (2) Use of BCP while breastfeeding
  - (a) Patient should be informed that a small amount of hormone from the pills passes through the milk to the baby. This amount of hormone is not considered to be dangerous by the American Academy of Pediatrics.
  - (b) There is potential suppression of the milk supply although this occurs less often on low-dose pills.
  - (c) Micronor or another progestin-only BCP are thought to have the least affect on breastfeeding.
- (3) Side effects and complications
  - (a) All major side effects, positive, negative, and common complications should be discussed with the patient. A consent form is recommended.
  - (b) Explain that any side effects she experiences will depend on how her particular body responds to the particular BCP she takes and that modifying the type of BCP will sometimes modify the side effects.
  - (c) Determine if she is taking any medications that would affect the hormone metabolism of BCP such as
    - i. Anticoagulants
    - ii. Aspirin
    - iii. Antibiotics, particularly penicillin and sulfa
    - iv. Antihistamines
    - v. Demerol
    - vi. Dilantin
    - vii. Rifampin
    - viii. Phenylbutazone
    - ix. Antidepressants, tranquilizers
  - (d) If patient has taken a particular BCP previously that she did well on, prescribe that kind when possible.
2. Instructions in starting the pill
   a. If patient is having menstrual cycles, have her take her first pill on the first Sunday or the fifth day after her next period starts.
   b. If patient is postpartum, start the pills on the second to sixth postpartum weeks to minimize the chance of thrombophlebitis. Caesarean section patients should be started at 6 weeks postpartum.
   c. If the patient is less than 12 weeks' postpartum but still amenorrheic due to lactation, she may start the pill anytime.
   d. If patient is postabortion (spontaneous or induced), start within 7 to 10 days.
3. Give the patient printed instructions that include

a. The importance of using an alternate method of contraception for the first month that BCPs are taken.
b. How to take the BCPs, including how to manage common errors in administration.
c. How to manage common side effects.
d. Which medications affect hormone metabolism and the importance of informing caregivers that she is on BCPs when drugs are prescribed.
e. When to call the office. Be sure patient is aware of the cardinal warning signs of BCP complications.
   (1) Severe abdominal pain: gallbladder or liver problem, embolism, pancreatitis
   (2) Severe chest pain or shortness of breath: pulmonary embolus or myocardial infarction
   (3) Severe headaches: stroke, hypertension, migraine
   (4) Eye problems: blurred vision, flashing lights, blindness
   (5) Severe leg pain (calf or thigh): thrombophlebitis
f. When to return for follow-up visit
g. Sign BCP consent form, offer a copy to the patient.

4. Follow-up
   a. Between the first 6 to 12 weeks of BCP usage, patient should be checked for the following:
      (1) Weight. An unexplained gain or loss of 10 pounds or more in 1 month requires further investigation.
      (2) Blood pressure. If abnormal, 140/90 or greater, and not on medication, needs close follow-up.
   b. Management of breakthrough bleeding
      (1) May resolve spontaneously within 3 months of taking the pills. Advise patient to wait unless very heavy bleeding noted.
      (2) If still present in fourth cycle after starting the pills, the pill needs to be switched:
         (a) Bleeding early in the cycle may be due to an estrogen deficiency. Change to pill with increased estrogen potency.
         (b) Bleeding late in the cycle may be due to estrogen or progesterone. Consult a text to determine which BCPs may eliminate this problem.
         (c) If on a triphasic BCP, switch to a monophasic BCP.
         (d) Ask patient about any side effects, questions, or concerns.
         (e) If any problems
            i. May try a different type of pill if etiology seems related to hormone dosage
            ii. Consult one of the many tables that show amount and potency of various BCPs
         (f) If all is well

i. Prescribe pills until 1 year or next Pap smear due.
ii. Be sure patient still has her printed instructions.
5. Management of amenorrhea:
    a. Anything, including brown spotting, is a period
    b. If patient is concerned about possible pregnancy, do a pregnancy test to confirm or rule out. If positive, provide pregnancy counseling.
    c. Try switching pills to another brand, preferably one with an increased estrogen effect.
    d. Add Estrace 1 to 2 mg or another estrogen days 1 to 21 of the BCPs for one to two cycles.

IX. Spermicides
   A. Definition: Chemical agents that inactivate the sperm in the vagina. Spermicides come in many forms from jellies, creams, and suppositories, to foams and thin film sheets that look like plastic wrap.
   B. Effectiveness: Failure rates of 20% to 30% per year are common.
   C. Advantages
      1. Can be bought over-the-counter
      2. Provide some protection against STDs, including HIV
      3. Low cost
   D. Disadvantages
      1. Require application 10 to 30 minutes before sexual intercourse
      2. Jellies, creams, and foam remain effective for 6 to 8 hours while suppositories lose effectiveness in 1 hour.
      3. Reapplication is necessary for each coital episode.
      4. Up to 5% of the population have an allergic response, which may be as mild as an unpleasant feeling, stinging, or increased discharge to major edema, pain, and the inability to urinate.
   E. Management
      1. Use with a condom is recommended to increase effectiveness
      2. Directions for each individual spermicide need to be read and followed exactly concerning time of insertion, length of effectiveness, and so on.

CARE DURING PREGNANCY

I. Philosophy
   A. Every childbearing family has a right to
      1. A safe, satisfying experience with respect for human dignity and worth
      2. Variety in cultural forms
      3. Self-determination

B. Comprehensive maternity care, including educational and emotional care throughout the childbearing years, is a major means for intercession into the improvement and maintenance of the health of the nation's families. Comprehensive maternity care is most effectively and efficiently delivered by interdependent health disciplines.[5]

II. **Objectives**
   A. To foster the delivery of safe, satisfying, and economical maternity care
   B. To recognize that childbearing is a family experience and encourage the active involvement of family members in the care process
   C. To uphold the right to self-determination of women and their families, within the boundaries of safe care
   D. To focus on health and growth as developmental processes during the reproductive years
   E. To use the reproductive experience as an opportunity to promote good health habits
   F. To stimulate community awareness and responsiveness to the need for alternatives in childbearing

III. **Initial Antepartum Visit**
   A. Purpose
      1. Conduct the initial visit, including a complete medical, OB, and family health history.
      2. Conduct a complete physical exam.
      3. Order and evaluate appropriate labwork and additional diagnostic procedures.
      4. Establish an estimated date of confinement.
      5. Identify deviations from the normal course of pregnancy.
      6. Delineate a plan of care, mutually agreed upon with the patient.
      7. Provide instruction and education to patients on the following topics related to normal pregnancy:
         a. Nutrition and weight gain
         b. Normal anatomic and physiologic changes
         c. Exercise and stress management
         d. Danger signs and when to contact the care provider
         e. Circumcision and preparation for the newborn
         f. Preparation for childbirth
         g. Sibling preparation for childbirth
         h. Family planning and contraception
         i. Preparation for breastfeeding
         j. Selection of a pediatrician
         k. Adjustment to family roles
         l. Referral to appropriate community services

---

[5]American College of Nurse-Midwives. 1990.

Care During Pregnancy   27

B. History: Initial history to be completed as outlined under gynecologic care. Also include in the OB history:
  1. Any exposure to the following:
     a. Tobacco, alcohol, caffeine, or saccharine
     b. Prescription or street drugs during pregnancy
     c. Aspirin or ibuprofen
     d. X-rays during pregnancy
     e. Extreme heat during pregnancy, such as fever, hot tubs, or saunas
     f. Toxoplasmosis
        (1) Exposure to cat feces by emptying the cat's litter box. This is most critical when the cat has access to wild birds or animals.
        (2) Eating rare or raw meat
     g. Primary herpes in first trimester and/or pattern of recurrent lesions or history of herpes genitalis
  2. Current pregnancy history
     a. Contraceptive use before this pregnancy
     b. First day of last *normal* menstrual period and any bleeding since then
     c. Signs and symptoms of pregnancy to date
     d. Date of positive pregnancy test
C. Physical exam: As outlined under gynecologic care. In addition:
  1. Abdominal exam
     a. Assess for progressive abdominal and uterine enlargement
     b. Measure fundal height
     c. Auscultate fetal heart tones
        (1) By doppler greater than 10 weeks' gestation
        (2) By fetoscope at 18 to 20 weeks' gestation for dating
     d. Assess fetal position (Leopold's maneuvers) after 28 weeks.
  2. Pelvic exam
     a. Observe for presumptive signs of pregnancy.
        (1) Chadwick's sign: a bluish coloring of the vulva and vaginal mucosa
        (2) Goodell's sign: softening of the cervix
        (3) Hegar's sign: softening and compressibility of the uterine isthmus
     b. If pregnancy is advanced, check for dilation and effacement.
     c. Evaluate pelvic type and size.
D. Labwork
  1. Initial labwork
     a. At the initial visit, all patients should have the following labwork done, unless they can produce evidence that it has been done elsewhere during the present pregnancy:
        (1) Complete blood count (CBC)
        (2) Serology

(3) Blood type and Rh factor
(4) Antibody titer
(5) Rubella titer
(6) Hepatitis B screen
(7) Urinalysis

    b. At the initial physical exam, a Pap smear, GC, and chlamydia culture should be done on all patients.

    c. Additional labwork may be ordered if indicated.

(1) HIV screen
(2) Sickle cell screen
(3) Beta-strep culture
(4) Herpes culture
(5) Thyroid screen
(6) Fasting blood sugar and 1-hour PP
(7) Clotting time, prothrombin time, partial thromboplastin time, platelet count, fibrinogen level
(8) Alpha-fetoprotein (AFP) or AFP-Plus at 15 to 18 weeks
(9) Wet mount

2. Routine labwork during the antepartum course includes:

    a. Dipstix of urine at each prenatal visit for

(1) Glucose
(2) Protein

    b. CBC and 1 hour post-glucola at 24 to 28 weeks

    c. Antibody titer on all Rh(D) negative patients at initial visit and at 24 to 28 weeks. If a patient registers for care after 30 weeks and has not received prophylactic RhoGAM, it is usually given until 36 weeks.

    d. For additional labwork that might be indicated, see Laboratory Tests on p. 41

E. Ultrasonography: Can be done if indicated. If only one is ordered, it is best done between 18 to 22 weeks. Indications for ordering include:

1. Unsure dates
2. Size/dates discrepancy
3. Question of abnormality

    a. Placenta previa
    b. Multiple gestation
    c. Fetal anomaly
    d. Maternal abnormality

IV. Return Antepartum Visit

A. Schedule for return visits

1. 1 to 28 weeks' gestation: every 4 weeks
2. 28 to 36 weeks' gestation: every 2 weeks
3. 36 weeks' gestation until term: every week

4. 41 weeks' gestation until birth: twice a week
   B. Teaching and counseling
      1. Provide opportunity for patient to discuss questions, concerns, and needs.
      2. Review checklist for topics to be discussed and procedures to be done at the appropriate weeks of gestation.
      3. Provide individualized health instruction, counseling, and guidance
      4. Review recent laboratory reports.
      5. Provide relief for minor discomforts or physical complaints.
      6. Referral for other needed services, for example:
         a. Dietitian
         b. Dentist or physician
         c. Social services or mental health services
         d. Childbirth education
         e. Physical therapist
      7. Formation and revision of plan of care after discussing options with patient
   C. Physical assessment
      1. Weeks gestation. Review dates if necessary. (See Establishing the Estimated Date of Confinement on p. 126.)
      2. Weight
      3. Blood pressure
      4. Fundal height
      5. Fetal heart rate
      6. Presenting part
      7. Urine dipstix for sugar and protein
      8. Vaginal exams are performed at the following times:
         a. The initial physical exam
         b. At 36 to 37 weeks if unsure of presentation
         c. At 40 weeks and beyond
         d. At other times as appropriate:
            (1) To check for labor
            (2) History of threatened premature labor
            (3) History of cone biopsy or other cervical surgery
            (4) Twin gestation—examine every 2 weeks after 24 weeks
            (5) Any other medical indication
            (6) At the patient's request as long as membranes are intact.
V. **Collaborative Care and Referral**
   A. Conditions that may be considered for collaborative management include:
      1. History of seizure disorder or epilepsy controlled by medication
      2. Two or more consecutive spontaneous abortions (see Abortion on p. 85)

3. More than five previous deliveries
4. Acute pyelonephritis or frequent UTI
5. Primipara over 35 years, or multipara aged 40 years or greater
6. Failure to gain weight
7. Abnormal presentation before labor
8. Postdates
9. Gestational diabetes
10. Prior fetal or neonatal death
11. Genital herpes
12. Uterine bleeding or history of postpartum hemorrhage
13. Polyhydramnios or oligohydramnios
14. Fetal growth retardation
15. Premature rupture of membranes over 12 hours without regular uterine contractions
16. Twin pregnancy
17. Alcohol and drug abuse
18. Anemia (hemoglobin less than 10, hematocrit less than 30%)
19. Positive PPD test for TB but negative chest radiograph
20. Uterine myomata
21. Pre-eclampsia
22. Asthma
23. Hypothyroidism
24. Hepatitis carrier
25. Pap smear of class III or greater
26. Persistent vomiting
27. Severe recurrent headaches
28. Absence of fetal heart tones and/or fetal movement after 28 weeks' gestation
29. Concern or request of patient to see a physician
30. Previous caesarean section

B. Conditions that necessitate referral to a physician include:
1. Previous classical caesarean section
2. Chronic hypertension, poorly controlled
3. Heart disease class II to IV
4. Active tuberculosis or other lung disease
5. Rh(D) negative with positive antibody titer
6. Hydatidiform mole
7. Renal disease, moderate to severe
8. Diabetes mellitus greater than class I
9. Hepatitis during pregnancy
10. Severe psychiatric disorders
11. Uncontrolled seizure disorder

12. Acute or chronic neurologic disorder
13. History of severe pre-eclampsia/eclampsia
14. Bleeding disorders
15. Placenta previa
16. Positive HIV

NUTRITION AND WEIGHT GAIN IN PREGNANCY

I. **Appropriate Weight Gain**
   A. Appropriate weight gain should be discussed at the initial OB visit.
   B. Determine normal weight for patient's height by using method below or any other weight/height table:
      1. One hundred pounds for the first 5 feet of height, add 5 pounds for every additional inch
      2. Small frame, subtract 10%
      3. Large frame, add 10%
   C. Determine patient's prepregnancy weight.
   D. Inform patient that she should gain 25 to 40 pounds, depending on her body build and prepregnancy weight.
   E. Take a diet history and do diet counseling.

II. **Good Nutrition Must Be Emphasized**
   A. Increased calorie needs
      1. Pregnancy: +300 calories
      2. Breastfeeding: +500 calories
   B. Daily: 80 to 100 gm of protein
      1. Reason
         a. To enable the body to lay down new tissue
         b. For fetal growth
         c. To prevent edema
      2. Foods
         a. 1 quart milk (32 gm)
         b. Three servings of meat, fish, chicken, rice, and beans (60–90 gm)
   C. Whole grains
      1. Reason
         a. Prevents constipation
         b. Good source of B vitamins
         c. Complex carbohydrate for energy
      2. Foods: Four servings of whole grain breads, pasta, cereals, legumes
   D. Milk and dairy products
      1. Reason
         a. Good source of protein and calcium

2. Foods:
   a. Four servings daily of low fat milk, cheese, cottage cheese
E. Fruits and vegetables
   1. Reasons
      a. Provides many vitamins and minerals
      b. Citrus high in vitamin C
      c. Helps prevent constipation
   2. Foods
      a. Five servings daily
      b. Make sure lettuce is dark green variety.
F. Water
   1. To keep up with expanding blood volume
   2. To avoid constipation
   3. Drink two quarts of fluid a day.
G. Twins
   1. Need an extra 30 gm of protein a day
   2. Need extra 200 calories a day
H. Substances to avoid
   1. Artificial sweeteners, especially Aspartame, which can be associated with headaches, dizziness
   2. Caffeine
   3. Drinks and foods with a high sugar content

III. **The Patient Should Be Weighed at Each Prenatal Visit.**
IV. **The Following Trends in Weight Gain Are Causes for Concern.**
   A. A weight loss at any time during pregnancy of greater than 5 pounds
   B. Failure to gain appropriately
      1. Failure to gain any weight for 1 month
      2. Failure to gain at least 10 pounds by 28 weeks, 15 pounds by 35 weeks, and 20 pounds at term
   C. Excessive weight gain
      1. A gain of more than 5 pounds in 1 month or more than 2 pounds in 1 week
      2. A gain of more than 20 pounds by 20 weeks
      3. A total weight gain of more than 40 pounds
V. **Management**
   A. Loss of weight or failure to gain appropriately: try to determine reason and treat accordingly.
      1. Nausea/vomiting
      2. Heartburn/lack of room in stomach
      3. Fear of gaining weight
         a. Counsel, reassure, explain distribution of weight gained during pregnancy.

b. Emphasize importance of weight gain, explore body image and acceptability of large body to patient/partner/others.
   c. Offer referral to dietitian and/or mental health counselor.
B. Excessive weight gain: try to determine reason and treat accordingly.
   1. Multiple gestation: suspect if sudden or continuous large gain, out of proportion to woman's body build and eating habits
   2. Diabetes
   3. Edema: check for other signs of pre-eclampsia.
   4. Idiosyncratic weight gain, for example, history of large weight gain with previous pregnancies, which was lost after delivery
   5. Uncontrolled intake of food
      a. Counsel on diet, explain that baby needs nutritious food in moderate amounts, not junk foods and fats.
      b. Stress the importance of regular exercise in controlling weight gain.
      c. If patient desires, she may join a self-help weight control group, such as Weight Watchers, TOPS, Overeaters Anonymous, and so forth. Give her a copy of the 1800-calorie diabetic diet to follow. If she loses weight on 1800 calories, increase to 2200 to 2400 calories until weight gain is within normal range.

CARE DURING LABOR AND DELIVERY

I. **Initial Assessment**
   A. Determine if the patient is in labor
      1. Uterine contractions
         a. Time of onset
         b. Intensity
         c. Frequency
         d. Duration
      2. Status of membranes
         a. If ruptured, time of rupture
         b. Color
         c. Amount of fluid
      3. Presence of show
         a. Amount
         b. Consistency
         c. Color (rule out frank bleeding)
      4. Quality of fetal movement
   B. Ascertain estimated date of confinement
   C. Review antepartum course.
   D. Review history.
      1. Family history
      2. Medical and surgical history

3. Past OB history
4. History of present pregnancy
E. Perform physical exam.
 1. Observe mother's reaction to labor.
 2. Note vital signs.
 3. Palpate abdomen for:
    a. Uterine contractions
    b. Fundal height
    c. Condition of abdominal wall
    d. Fetus
       (1) Position
       (2) Presentation
       (3) Attitude
       (4) Estimated fetal weight
 4. Monitor fetal heart rate.
 5. Perform pelvic evaluation.
    a. Cervical dilation and effacement
    b. Fetal presentation, position of presenting part, and station
    c. Status of membranes
 6. Perform speculum exam as indicated for
    a. Diagnosis of spontaneous rupture of membranes
    b. Culture of cervix
    c. Visualization of vagina and cervix for any lesions (ie, history of herpes)
    d. Identification of source of vaginal bleeding

II. **Ongoing Management**
A. First stage of labor
 1. Observe and guide the physical progress of labor and birth.
 2. Continue assessment of labor.
    a. Monitor maternal blood pressure and temperature per guidelines.
    b. Evaluate uterine contractions for frequency, duration, and intensity.
    c. Perform cervical exams for dilation, effacement, station, and position of fetus.
    d. Monitor fetal heart rate for 20 minutes or through three contractions initially, then for 10 minutes or through two contractions every hour.
    e. Vaginal exams as necessary to assess labor. Limit with ruptured membranes.
 3. Ambulation will facilitate labor. Do **not** ambulate if membranes are ruptured and vertex is high.

4. Encourage hydration either through oral or intravenous (IV) fluids. IV infusion is necessary for
   a. Clinical signs of dehydration
   b. Prolonged vomiting and/or inability to drink or retain oral fluids
5. Heparin lock or TKO IV is indicated for the following:
   a. Greater than para V
   b. Hemoglobin and hematocrit below 9.0 and 27%, respectively.
   c. History of bleeding disorder or previous postpartum hemorrhage
   d. Breech presentation
   e. Twin gestation
   f. Hypertension or other medical conditions
6. Amniotomy
   a. Indications
      (1) To induce labor
      (2) To stimulate labor
      (3) To check for presence of meconium if fetal distress or maternal complications, such as hypertension, prolonged labor, and so on
   b. Criteria
      (1) Vertex presentation with head at -2 station or lower
      (2) Term pregnancy
      (3) Cervix ripe, with Bishop's score of at least 8 (a score of 9 is almost fail-proof)
7. Provide pain relief as desired by the patient and according to approved guidelines.
8. Assist the patient and her family to cope with labor and birth by providing support and comfort measures.
9. Identify deviations from normal.
   a. Manage frequently encountered problems according to approved guidelines.
   b. Consult or refer when indicated.
10. Document progress of labor, deviations from normal, and any consultations.

B. Second stage of labor
1. Teach the patient proper bearing-down technique.
2. Provide emotional support.
3. Auscultate fetal heart rate every 5 minutes or with continuous electronic monitoring.
4. Catheterization is necessary if bladder is distended and patient is unable to void.
5. Conduct single vertex normal spontaneous vaginal delivery.

6. Participate in twin, breech, and premature delivery with appropriate physician collaboration.
7. Perform episiotomy if needed.
8. Perform immediate appraisal of newborn, assign Apgar scores, and consult with physician or neonatal nurse practitioner as indicated.

C. Third stage of labor
1. Deliver and inspect placenta, cord, and membranes.
2. Collect cord blood for type, Rh, Venereal Disease Research Laboratory (VDRL), and HIV, as required.
3. Collect cord blood for gases if non-reassuring fetal heart rate pattern, terminal bradycardia, difficult delivery. Send to lab if 1-minute Apgar score is 5 or below.
4. Control postpartum bleeding by massage of the fundus and use of oxytocic drugs if needed.
5. Culture placenta if prolonged rupture of membranes or fever.
6. Perform perineal, vaginal, and cervical inspection.
7. Perform local infiltration or pudendal block anesthesia if needed.
8. Repair perineal, vaginal, and cervical lacerations or episiotomy.
9. Promote early infant-parent contact and breastfeeding.

D. Medication: The nurse-midwife may order the following:
1. Phenergan 25 to 50 mg IM or IV every 3 to 4 hours as necessary for relief of anxiety or nausea
2. Vistaril 50 to 100 mg IM only, every 3 to 4 hours as necessary for relief of anxiety or nausea
3. Stadol 1 to 2 mg every 2 to 4 hours as necessary for pain
4. Demerol 25 to 50 mg IM or IV every 3 to 4 hours as necessary for pain, after active labor is well established
5. Morphine sulfate 10 to 15 mg IM to stop latent labor and permit rest
6. A hypnotic such as Seconal or Nembutal 100 mg orally to take home for sedation in latent labor

E. Postpartum care
1. In hospital
   a. Manage patient's hospital course.
      (1) Fourth stage of labor
         (a) Vital signs
         (b) Estimated blood loss and current lochia flow
         (c) Fundus for consistency and location
         (d) Bladder status
         (e) Condition of genital area
         (f) Status of hydration and nutrition
         (g) Psychosocial status
         (h) Maternal–infant bonding

- (2) Order appropriate labwork.
  - (a) Hemoglobin and hematocrit 12 to 24 hours after delivery
  - (b) Cultures as indicated (see Puerperal Infection on page 212)
    - i. Endocervical
    - ii. Urine
    - iii. Blood
  - (c) Other labwork as indicated
- (3) Visit patient daily while hospitalized.
  - (a) Review history and progress to date.
  - (b) Perform daily physical exam, to include:
    - i. Breasts and nipples
    - ii. Abdomen and uterus
    - iii. Lochia
    - iv. Vulva and perineum
    - v. Costovertebral angle tenderness
    - vi. Extremities (Homans's sign)
  - (c) Provide postpartum instruction
- **b.** Foster family bonding and adjustment to the newborn.
- **c.** Identify deviations from the normal puerperium.
  - (1) Manage frequently encountered problems according to approved guidelines.
  - (2) Consult or refer when indicated.
- **d.** Identify patient's informational needs and instruct regarding:
  - (1) Normal anatomic and physiologic changes
  - (2) Nutrition and weight loss
  - (3) Exercise and activities
  - (4) Hygiene
  - (5) Danger signs and when to seek help
  - (6) Community resources for newborn care
  - (7) Breastfeeding or lactation suppression
  - (8) Sexuality and contraception
  - (9) Referral to appropriate community resources
- **e.** Obtain relevant laboratory tests.
- **f.** Assist in planning home care.
- **g.** Keep adequate hospital records according to standard chart forms. Chart progress notes on any events out of the ordinary.
- **h.** Discharge patients from the hospital if:
  - (1) No medical problems requiring close supervision (eg, high blood pressure, diabetes)
  - (2) No antepartum or intrapartum OB complications requiring close postpartum observation (eg, hemorrhage, infection,)

    (3) Asymptomatic with hemoglobin and hematocrit equal to or above 9.0 and 27%, respectively
    (4) Baby has been released by pediatrician or family practice physician
2. In office (4 to 8 weeks postpartum)
    a. Evaluate physical and emotional condition of mother.
        (1) History
            (a) Review antepartum and intrapartum course.
            (b) General health of the mother: weight loss or gain, rest, fatigue
            (c) Family and mother's adjustment to newborn
            (d) Breastfeeding
            (e) Amount and type of lochia
            (f) Resumption of sexual relations and any problems
            (g) Emotional state
        (2) Physical exam
            (a) Blood pressure, pulse, weight
            (b) Auscultate heart and lungs.
            (c) Examine breasts for nipple integrity, masses, inflammation, engorgement.
            (d) Palpate abdomen for tenderness, masses, involution of the uterus, and diastis recti.
            (e) Examine legs for indications of thrombophlebitis.
            (f) Examine external genitalia for lesions, healing of episiotomy or lacerations, abnormalities of the Bartholin's and Skene's glands.
            (g) Perform speculum exam. Note lacerations of cervix, discharge, lesions. Obtain specimen for Pap smear.
            (h) Perform bimanual exam. Check for any abnormalities of cervix, uterus, adnexae, state of involution, presence of cystocele or rectocele, and vaginal muscle tone.
        (3) Provide mother with the opportunity to discuss any problems concerning baby, family, or herself.
        (4) Observe mother—infant interaction if baby is present.
        (5) Initiate a contraceptive method if desired.
        (6) Provide appropriate teaching.
            (a) Explain results of exam and necessity of yearly gynecologic exams.
            (b) Encourage regular aerobic, abdominal, and Kegel exercises.
            (c) Counsel on choice of contraceptive method.
            (d) Explain the benefits of a good diet and vitamins.
            (e) Discuss course of breastfeeding.

III. **Consultation and/or Collaborative Management**
   A. Consultation and/or collaborative management with a physician is appropriate for the following situations:
      1. Vaginal birth after caesarean section
      2. Premature or prolonged rupture of membranes
      3. Abnormal presentation
      4. Abnormal vaginal bleeding
      5. Twin pregnancy
      6. Polyhydramnios or oligohydramnios
      7. Hypertension
      8. Diabetes mellitus, class I
      9. Prolonged active labor: no progress for 3 hours with a questionable contraction pattern or no progress for 2 hours with an adequate contraction pattern.
      10. Prolonged second stage: no progress for 1 hour or a second stage lasting longer than 2 hours.
      11. Preterm labor—37 weeks or less
      12. Cord prolapse
      13. Fetal distress
         a. Extended bradycardia or tachycardia
         b. Multiple late or variable decelerations
         c. Non-reassuring fetal heart rate pattern
      14. Postterm—Over 42 weeks
      15. Other maternal or fetal distress
      16. Inappropriate gestational size
      17. Signs of genital herpes
      18. Moderately or heavily meconium-stained amniotic fluid
      19. Abnormalities immediately after delivery
         a. Retained placenta
         b. Postpartum hemorrhage that does not respond to the following measures:
            (1) Oxytocic drugs
            (2) Fundal massage, bimanual compression, or both
            (3) Supine position
            (4) Rapid administration of IV fluids
            (5) Oxygen per mask
   B. Referral to physician care is required in the following situations:
      1. Multiple pregnancy of greater than two fetuses
      2. Severe pre-eclampsia or eclampsia
      3. Diabetes mellitus greater than class I

4. Caesarean section (maternal or fetal indication) with a documented classical uterine incision

IV. Oxytocin Induction or Augmentation
   A. Admission procedures
      1. Be sure prenatal record and indication for procedure are on hospital chart.
      2. Take a brief history, including onset of labor, status of membranes, and presence of bleeding.
      3. Conduct a brief physical exam according to the standard form on the hospital chart.
      4. Indicate selection of standing orders and sign.
      5. Labwork
         a. Complete blood count
         b. Clot tube to be held
         c. Type and screen only if high likelihood of hemorrhage and surgery
   B. Induction
      1. Indications
         a. Postdates
         b. Premature rupture of membranes
         c. Polyhydramnios or oligohydramnios
         d. Fetal indications
            (1) Nonreactive nonstress test
            (2) Biophysical profile below 8
            (3) Large for gestational age
            (4) Suspected intrauterine fetal growth retardation.
      2. Criteria
         a. Patient must be greater than 37 weeks' estimated gestational age.
         b. Prior consultation with back-up physician
      3. Method
         a. Amniotomy
         b. Prostaglandin gel or Prepidil per hospital protocol
            (1) Unripe cervix
            (2) Bishop's score of 4 or below, with or without ruptured membranes (see Table 3–5 on pg. 199)
         c. Pitocin per hospital protocol
   C. Augmentation
      1. Indications
         a. Rupture of membranes without active labor
         b. Poor uterine contractions
         c. Failure to progress with active labor; cervix unchanged in 3 hours in primiparous or 2 hours in the multiparous patient

2. Criteria
   a. Vertex presentation
   b. Reassuring fetal heart rate pattern
   c. Physician consultation
D. Management (see section on Ongoing Management on page 34)

LABORATORY STUDIES

I. **Initial Prenatal Labwork:** Includes CBC with differential, blood type and Rh factor, antibody titer, serology, rubella titer, chlamydia, and GC. Optional tests include HIV, hepatitis panel, and TB.
   A. CBC with differential
      1. Ordered routinely at the initial prenatal visit
         a. If hemoglobin less than 11 and/or hematocrit less than 33, treat with extra iron and foods high in iron.
         b. If any other abnormal values, repeat lab if necessary to confirm and consult if needed.
      2. Order if any sign of systemic infection or bleeding.
   B. Hematocrit and hemoglobin: Assess as part of CBC at initial visit and at 26 to 28 weeks lab.
   C. Blood type and Rh factor
      1. Order for all pregnant patients at the initial visit.
         a. Antibody titer
            (1) If positive, has she had RhoGAM?
            (2) Repeat for antibody identification. Consult if the factor may be harmful to the fetus.
      2. Repeat antibody titer at 26 to 28 weeks' gestation for all Rh(D) negative patients.
      3. Give RhoGAM prophylactically to all Rh(D)–negative pregnant patients at 28 to 30 weeks' gestation. No further antibody screen need be done. If a patient has not previously received prophylactic RhoGAM, it may be given until 36 weeks.
   D. Serology
      1. Rapid plasma reagin (RPR)
         a. Ordered for all pregnant patients unless previous record of negative RPR or VDRL during present pregnancy. If positive, order fluorescent treponemal antibody absorption. (See Syphilis on page 232 for information on treatment.)
      2. VDRL
         a. Order VDRL if patient is diagnosed as having gonorrhea or chlamydia.
         b. VDRL is a titer which can become positive through infection by any number of febrile diseases as well as syphilis. Once the VDRL, RPR, or fluorescent treponemal antibody absorption become positive, they remain positive for life. The RPR is more

sensitive than the VDRL and therefore is useful for diagnosis of early syphilis, but only if the patient was previously RPR-negative. If previously positive, diagnosis **must be made on the basis of rising VDRL titers. A fourfold increase in titer indicates an active infection.** May need serial titers to confirm or rule out.

    c. After treatment, order follow-up VDRL monthly while pregnant, and at 3, 6, and 12 months. If the syphilis infection was of greater than 1-year duration, repeat VDRL 24 months after treatment.

E. Rubella titer
1. Order for all pregnant patients at initial visit.
2. If negative titer less than 1:10 IV/mL, recommend immunization after delivery.
3. If titer greater than 1:1000, repeat to rule out lab error.
    a. If still elevated, repeat in 3 weeks for potential convalescent serum.
    b. If decreased, consult concerning possible rubella in pregnancy.
4. If negative and possible exposure during pregnancy, may get serial titers.

F. Sickle cell screen
1. Order for all pregnant African American patients.
2. If positive, order hemoglobin electrophoresis.
    a. If homozygous, the patient has sickle cell disease. Refer to physician for care.
    b. If heterozygous, consider ordering electrophoresis to test the blood of the baby's father. If he is heterozygous, there is a chance that the baby could inherit sickle cell disease.

G. Hepatitis B screen
1. Order at the initial visit.
2. Obtain at any time during the pregnancy if clinical picture is suggestive. Consider if persistent nausea and vomiting, malaise, pruritus, jaundice.
3. If positive, see Hepatitis guidelines on page 147.

H. Serum alpha-fetoprotein (AFP) or AFP-Plus
1. AFP at 15 to 18 weeks' gestation
2. Offer AFP-Plus if:
    a. Patient is going to be 35 or over at the time of delivery and does not want amniocentesis.
    b. Patient had a previous child with a neural tube defect or Down's syndrome.
    c. Patient has a close relative who had a child with a neural tube defect or Down's syndrome.
    d. Patient was exposed to a temperature of 102°F or greater in the first trimester.

3. If positive, there may be an increased risk of a baby with a neural tube defect or Down's syndrome.
    a. Check estimated date of confinement with an ultrasound. If lab was drawn between 15 to 20 weeks' gestation, recalculate alpha-fetoprotein using corrected estimated gestational age (EGA). If lab not drawn at correct time, redraw alpha-fetoprotein when gestational age is correct.
    b. If risk remains elevated, refer for genetic counseling and possible amniocentesis.
I. Urinalysis and urine culture and sensitivity
    1. Order for all patients at initial visit and 26 to 28 weeks.
    2. If no history of frequent UTI and initial culture is positive, treat and repeat culture for test of cure following medication.
    3. If history of frequent UTI:
        a. With an initial negative culture, repeat culture at 27 to 28 weeks.
        b. Initial culture positive, treat and repeat culture 1 week after treatment and at 24 and 32 weeks.
    4. If signs and symptoms of UTI develop at any time during pregnancy, order a urinalysis and urine culture & sensitivity.
    5. If frequent UTIs during pregnancy:
        a. Consider screening for:
            (1) G6PD anemia if patient is African American, Asian, or of Mediterranean descent
            (2) Diabetes
        b. May need tests of kidney function, such as blood urea nitrogen, creatinine, 24-hour urinary creatinine clearance
        c. May need prophylactic treatment, such as Macrodantin 50 mg, one orally every day until delivered, if treated two or more times this pregnancy
    6. Urine test results that indicate UTI:
        a. Culture & sensitivity bacteria colony count greater than 100,000
        b. Clean-catch urinalysis
            (1) Bacteria
            (2) Nitrates
            (3) Red blood cells
            (4) May be proteinuria secondary to bacteriuria
            (5) White blood cells greater than 50/ml or greater than 25 per HPF spun urine
J. Dipstix urine test
    1. Performed at each prenatal visit
    2. If positive for ketones, review food intake.
    3. If positive glucose greater than +2 twice, see Diabetes guidelines on page 102.

4. If more than a trace protein:
   a. Obtain clean-catch or catheterized urine and recheck.
   b. If still present, rule out pre-eclampsia and pregnancy-induced hypertension.
   c. If no hypertension, obtain urine culture & sensitivity to rule out asymptomatic UTI.
   d. If no UTI, order kidney function tests, consult as necessary.
5. If positive for blood:
   a. Obtain a clean-catch or catheterized urine.
   b. If urine remains positive for more than a trace of blood, consult; may indicate a kidney stone or other problems.

K. Pap smear
   1. Annual Pap smear is recommended.
   2. Perform on all pregnant patients at new OB exam, unless one is documented within 6 months of exam.
   3. Perform on all patients presenting for exam who have not had one within a year.

L. Gonorrhea culture
   1. Perform at new OB exam.
   2. Perform at any time during pregnancy that patient presents with:
      a. Signs and symptoms
      b. Concern that she might have an STD
      c. Diagnosed with another STD
   3. If positive:
      a. Order VDRL and perform a chlamydia culture if not already done.
      b. Recommended treatment while pregnant is Rocephin 250 mg IM plus erythromycin 500 mg orally four times a day for 7 days.[6]
      c. Repeat culture
         (1) One week after treatment
         (2) At 36 weeks if treated during pregnancy
         (3) At the 6 weeks' postpartum visit if treated during pregnancy
   4. If still positive after treatment:
      a. Retreat.
      b. Re-instruct patient regarding importance of taking all medicine, mode of transmission, getting partner(s) treated, abstaining from intercourse until patient and partner have a negative culture.

M. Chlamydia culture
   1. Obtain on all new OB patients and also if:
      a. Clinical picture is suggestive of chlamydia
      b. Patient is diagnosed as having syphilis or gonorrhea

---

[6]Centers for Disease Control and Prevention. 1989.

2. If positive and pregnant, treat with amoxicillin 500 mg three times a day for 7 days.[7] Zithromax 1 gm orally or Zithromax cocktail is preferred by some because it is a one-dose treatment. At present, it is expensive. Repeat culture 2 to 3 weeks after treatment. If still positive:
   a. Retreat.
   b. Re-instruct patient regarding importance of taking all medicine, mode of transmission, getting partner(s) treated, abstaining from intercourse until patient and partner have a negative culture.
3. Notify pediatrician at delivery.

N. Herpes simplex culture
   1. Obtain any time suggestive lesions appear or if Pap smear suggestive of herpes is obtained.
   2. If positive or has history of herpes, see Herpes Simplex Virus guidelines on page 152.

O. Thyroid screen
   1. Obtain thyroid-stimulating hormone if:
      a. Patient has been on thyroid medication
      b. Any abnormality of the thyroid on exam
      c. Signs and/or symptoms of thyroid disease
   2. If abnormal results, perform thyroid panel and consult as necessary.

P. Blood sugar tests
   1. Obtain fasting blood sugar and 2-hour postprandial blood sugar or a 1-hour post 50 g glucola load.
      a. Preferably between 24 and 28 weeks
      b. Check institution/office guidelines to see if a 3-day high-glucose diet is required before this test.
      c. Do immediately if:
         (1) History of stillborn or unexplained neonatal death
         (2) History of gestational diabetes
         (3) Sibling or parent with insulin-dependent diabetes
         (4) Two consecutive episodes of glycosuria unrelated to carbohydrate intake
         (5) Strong suspicion of diabetes, based on two or more predisposing factors
   2. If any of the values obtained are abnormal, obtain a 3-hour GTT. Results are considered abnormal if the following values are met or exceeded:
      a. Fasting blood sugar greater than 105 mg glucose/100 ml plasma
      b. Two-hour postprandial greater than 140
      c. One-hour post 50 g glucola greater than 140.

---

[7]Centers for Disease Control and Prevention. 1989.

d. If more than 200, a presumptive diagnosis of gestational diabetes is made. A 3-hour GTT need not be done. See Gestational Diabetes Management on page 103.
 e. GTT upper limits
  (1) Fasting blood sugar 105
  (2) One-half or one-hour 195
  (3) Two-hour 165
  (4) Three-hour 145
 3. If any two GTT values are above normal, see Diabetes guidelines on page 103.
Q. Clotting time, PT, PTT, platelet count, fibrinogen level
 1. Obtain if:
  a. History of abnormal clotting, severe anemia and/or unusually long or heavy menstrual periods
  b. Platelet count less than 100 on CBC
  c. Potential disseminated intravascular coagulation. (See Bleeding in Pregnancy Over 20 Weeks' Gestation on page 89.)
 2. Consult with physician if abnormal results.
R. Wet mount; obtain if:
 1. Unusual or suspicious discharge seen on routine exam
 2. Patient complains of vaginal discharge and/or itching, burning, irritation.
S. Cervical culture; obtain if:
 1. Abortion threatened or complete
 2. Prolonged rupture of membranes
 3. Endometritis
 4. History of premature labor and/or previous vaginal beta-strep
T. Stool for ova and parasites: obtain if:
 1. Diarrhea, unrelieved for 48 hours despite treatment
 2. Severe anemia or anemia that does not respond to treatment. Also obtain guaiac.
U. Serum pregnancy test
 1. To determine pregnancy
 2. Preoperative
 3. Serial quantitative beta human chorionic gonadotropin (QBHCG) test can be ordered every 2 to 3 days to check the viability of fetus.

II

Common Discomforts of Pregnancy

Discomfort	Etiology	Differential Diagnosis	Relief Measures	Danger Signs
Back pain, lower	1. Muscle strain caused by shift in the center of gravity caused by enlarging uterus. 2. High blood levels of progesterone softens cartilage & loosens stable pelvic joints allowing movement. 3. Lax abdominal muscle tone, especially in multiparas.	1. Uterine contractions. 2. Genital infections. 3. UTIs. 4. Sciatica. 5. Herniated disk. 6. Vertebral tumor. 7. Muscle sprain or strain. 8. Kidney infection or disease.	1. Wear maternity support girdle. 2. Take warm tub baths. 3. Firm supportive mattress may be helpful & assume lateral recumbent position with pillows supporting back & legs. 4. Use local head and back rubs. 5. Use relaxation techniques. 6. Avoid excessive twisting, bending, stretching, also excessive standing or walking. 7. Use proper body mechanics, pelvic tilt and other exercises to strenghthen back; refer to physical therapist for such. 8. Exercise program encourages general fitness. 9. When standing for long periods, rest one foot on low stool, & when sitting for long periods, rest feet on low stool, raise knees above the waist, & sit with back firmly against back of chair. 10. When driving, sit straight with knees slightly bent when using pedals. 11. Maintain good posture & wear shoes with 2-inch heels 12. Tylenol 650 mg every 4 hr; PRN minor discomfort.	History of back injury, or other back problems, surgery, UTI symptoms, ruptured membranes, uterine contractions, neurologic deficit, CVAT, pain with straight-leg raises, abnormal DTRs, abnormal vaginal discharge.

(continued)

(Continued)

Discomfort	Etiology	Differential Diagnosis	Relief Measures	Danger Signs
Back pain, upper	1. Muscle strain caused by shift in the center of gravity, caused by enlarging uterus. 2. High blood levels of progesterone soften cartilage & loosen stable pelvic joints. 3. Increased breast size.	1. Uterine contractions. 2. Kidney infection or disease. 3. UTIs. 4. Sciatica. 5. Herniated disk. 6. Vertebral tumor. 7. Muscle sprain or strain. 8. Gallbladder disease.	1. Wear good, supportive bra. 2. Take warm tub baths. 3. Firm supportive mattress may be helpful & assume lateral recumbent position with pillows supporting back & legs. 4. Use local heat and back rubs. 5. Use relaxation techniques. 6. Avoid excessive twisting, bending, & stretching, also excessive walking or standing. 7. Use exercises to strengthen back; refer to physical therapist for such. 8. Exercise program encourages general fitness. 9. Maintain good posture. 10. Tylenol 650 mg every 4 hr; PRN minor discomfort.	History of back injury or other back problems, surgery, UTI symptoms, ruptured membranes, uterine contractions, neurologic deficit, CVAT, pain with straight-leg raises, abnormal DTRs, abnormal vaginal discharge.
Constipation	1. Increased progesterone levels in pregnancy cause relaxation of smooth muscle of bowel, resulting in decreased motility, tone, and peristalsis of the GI tract.	1. Preterm labor. 2. Irritable bowel syndrome. 3. Appendicitis. 4. Intestinal obstruction. 5. Fecal obstruction.	1. Dietary changes—increase roughage and fluids (fresh fruits and vegetables, dried fruits, bran, whole grain foods, drink 6–8 glasses of liquids daily, hot drink on arising). 2. Increase exercise. 3. Maintain regular bowel habits.	Changes in stool, diarrhea, abdominal pain, fever, anorexia, periumbilical pain, rectal bleeding, emotional distress, or excessive laxative use for weight control.

	2. Large bowel is mechanically compressed by enlarging uterus. 3. Changes in food & fluid intake or exercise level due to pregnancy changes. 4. Prenatal vitamins with iron or calcium.	4. If taking prenatal vitamins, use one with stool softener. 5. If needed, take nonsystemic bulk laxative stool softener or combination of softener & laxative. 6. If acute, try Ducolax, MOM, or glycerine suppository. 7. If all else fails, try Fleets enema. Do not use acute measures regularly.	
Dependent edema	1. High estrogen levels may make blood vessels more fragile and "leaky." 2. Impaired venous circulation and increased pressure in lower extremities from pressure of enlarging uterus on veins. 3. May be due to expanding blood volume of pregnancy.	1. Avoid constrictive clothing. 2. Take rest periods lying down on left side with legs elevated periodically throughout day to aid venous return. 3. Elastic stocking may aid venous return. 4. Avoid excessive sodium. 5. Call if edema suddenly becomes more severe or general.	Sudden onset or generalization (facial or upper extremity) may be sign of PIH. Numbness or loss of sensation in fingers of either or both hands. Confusion, headache, flashing lights, fatigue, N & V, dyspnea, upper abdominal pain, decreased fetal movement, decreased urine output, rapid weight gain (more than 2 lb/wk), in-
	1. PIH—usually more severe than physiologic with sudden onset and more generalized. 2. High sodium intake—sodium should not be restricted during pregnancy, but consuming excessive amount may result in edema. 3. HELLP syndrome, renal disease, varicosities, local trauma to extremities, Car-		

(continued)

(Continued)

Discomfort	Etiology	Differential Diagnosis	Relief Measures	Danger Signs
Dependent edema (*continued*)		pal tunnel syndrome, & congestive heart failure.		crease in BP of 30 mm Hg systolic or 15 mmHg diastolic over baseline.
Dyspareunia	1. Pressure from enlarging uterus. 2. Inflammation. 3. Anatomic abnormalities. 4. Pelvic pathology. 5. Atrophy. 6. Failure of lubrication. 7. History of STDs. 8. Recurrent infection. 9. Psychological conflicts.	1. Vulvovaginitis. 2. Atrophic vulvovaginitis. 3. Hymenal strands. 4. Scar tissue. 5. Episiotomy. 6. Vaginismus. 7. Pelvic relaxation. 8. PID. 9. Pelvic masses. 10. Bartholin's cyst. 11. Inappropriate sexual technique. 12. Psychological factors, such as previous sexual trauma, stress.	1. Try to alternate positions during intercourse. 2. Use water-soluble lubricant. 3. Refer to psychological therapy if appropriate. 4. Explore alternate methods to express intimacy & affection. 5. Take medication for inflammation & infection, if appropriate.	Uterine contractions, vulvar &/or vaginal inflammation, lesions, discharge, pelvic masses (other than pregnancy), cervical motion tenderness, loss of pelvic support, symptoms of UTI.
Fatigue	Occurs primarily during first & third trimesters. 1. 1st trimester—increased oxygen	Fatigue can be a symptom in most pathological problems—emotional, physical, or dietary.	1. Increased fatigue is expected in first & third trimester. 2. Verbal psychosocial problems & seek apt interventions. 3. Accept offers of help.	History of depression, anxiety, difficulty with concentration, anorexia, anemia, exercise intolerance, chest pain or dis-

	Etiology	Management	Signs/Follow-up
	consumption, progesterone levels, & fetal demands; psychosocial changes. 2. Third trimester—sleep disturbances from increased weight, physical discomforts, & decreased exercise.	4. Avoid, if possible, major life stresses during pregnancy. 5. Take supplemental iron if anemic. 6. Get adequate sleep; take rest periods, maintain good posture; wear low-heeled shoes; perform pelvic rock exercises. 8. Correct nutritional inadequacies. 9. Avoid caffeine & heavy meals at end of day.	comfort, change in bowel habits, flu-liky symptoms, sore throat, coughing or dyspnea, or other symptoms/signs indicating other conditions requiring medical or other follow-up. Abnormal vital signs or lab work, especially CBC.
Gas	Increased progesterone levels in pregnancy cause relaxation of smooth muscle of bowel, resulting in decreased motility, tone, and peristalsis of the GI tract.	1. Irritable bowel syndrome. 2. Lactose intolerance. 3. Medication side effects. 4. Hyperventilation. 1. Learn measures to avoid constipation. 2. Learn symptoms of hyperventilation or air swallowing. 3. Avoid gum chewing, large meals, & smoking. 4. Limit gas-forming foods (carbonated beverages, cheese, beans, bananas, calcium carbonate supplements). 5. Take Phazyme.	Changes in bowel habits, dark, tarry stools, grey, mucousy stools, abdominal pain, &/or tenderness.
Headache	1. Increased circulatory volume. 2. Vasodilation from high levels of circulating progesterone.	1. Tension, migraine, cluster, sinus, or benign vascular HA. 2. PIH. 1. Keep diary of activites, foods, & environmental stimuli that occur around time of HA. 2. Learn symptoms of PIH. 3. Acetaminophen 325–650 mg every 4 hrs; PRN pain.	History of injury to head, neck, or back; occupational exposure to chemicals; consumption of al- *(continued)*

54 Part II: Common Discomforts of Pregnancy

(Continued)

Discomfort	Etiology	Differential Diagnosis	Relief Measures	Danger Signs
Headache (*continued*)	3. Tissue edema resulting from vascular congestion. 4. Stress. 5. Fatigue. 6. Low blood sugar.	3. URI or sinus infection. 4. Fever. 5. Cardiovascular disease. 6. Cervical arthritis. 7. Muscle tension HA. 8. Cerebellar mass or hemorrhage. 9. CNS infection. 10. Hypoglycemia.	4. Avoid activities & situations that may trigger HA. 5. Reduce stress as much as possible, get adequate sleep, have neck & shoulders massaged with heat or coolness applied. 6. Practice relaxation techniques. 7. Eat regular, balanced diet & avoid intake of food that triggers HA. 8. Refer to pain center if pain unrelieved by these measures or counseling.	cohol, chocolate, or aged cheese; unbalanced intake of calories; or fatigue—these S/S may indicate conditions requiring follow-up. History of facial edema, changes in level of consciousness, memory changes, motor visual, or sensory changes, N & V, stiff neck, fever, ear or eye pain, rhinitis, flu-like symptoms, injury. Urine dipstick with more than trace protein or ketones, low serum glucose, abnormal CBC.
Heartburn	1. Increase in levels of circulating progesterone that causes decreased	1. Cardiac. 2. Gallbladder. 3. Epigastric, or pancreatic disease.	1. This is related to pregnancy and should improve or disappear after pregnancy. 2. Do not lie down, bend, or stoop	Chest pain, shortness of breath, exercise intolerance, palpitations, sweating, anx-

| | peristalsis and relaxation of hiatal sphincter.
2. Pressure of gravid uterus against intestines and stomach increases the reflux of gastric contents into esophagus. | 4. Gastroenteritis or hiatal disease. | for 2 hr after eating.
3. Elevate head of bed 6 in.
4. Avoid clothing that constricts around abdomen or waist.
5. Stop smoking.
6. Avoid hot, spicy, fatty, gas-forming foods, coffee, alcohol, & gum chewing.
7. Eat small, frequent meals & chew throroughly.
8. Avoid excessive weight gain.
9. Antacids (Maalox, Mylanta, Pepcid AC) to relieve hyperacidity and gas; if contain aluminum & magnesium hydroxide, iron absorption may be impaired, so take iron & vitamin supplements at least 2 hr before or after taking antacids.
10. Use calcium carbonate with caution, may cause rebound hyperacidity.
11. Avoid sodium bicarbonate. | iety, upper abdominal pain (especially after heavy, fatty, or spicy meals), fatty, foul-smelling stools, N & V, fever or flu-like symptoms. |
| **Hemorrhoids** | 1. Impaired venous circulation with resulting congestion in pelvic veins.
2. Increased venous pressure on pelvic veins due to pressure of enlarging uterus. | 1. Abscessed or thrombosed hemorrhoids.
2. Cancerous lesions.
3. Idiopathic pruritis ani.
4. Condyloma acuminata.
5. Rectal fissure. | 1. Physician will examine for severity, trauma & possible thrombosis—if thrombosed, will refer to surgeon for lancing.
2. If no improvement after 1 wk, physician will re-examine for trauma or thrombosis.
3. Comfort measures: *a.* review diet & modify to keep stools soft; *b.* relieve constipation; *c.* frequent sitz | Decreased hemoglobin due to prolonged or extensive bleeding. Severe pain, blue-black in color, thrombosis. |

(continued)

(Continued)

Discomfort	Etiology	Differential Diagnosis	Relief Measures	Danger Signs
Hemorrhoids (*continued*)	3. Relaxing effects of progesterone on vein walls and valves. 4. Constipation. 5. Straining at stool. 6. Family tendency.		baths; *d.* ice packs, witch hazel packs, & Epsom salt compresses to reduce swelling; *e.* rubber ring to sit on for reduction of pressure; *f.* keep reduced by gently pushing hemorrhoids inside the rectum & tightening the rectal sphincter to give them support & to contain them within rectum; *g.* bed rest with hips & lower extremities elevated; *h.* medical suppositories, Preparation H, topical analgesic/anesthetic spray or ointment if needed; and *i.* if bleeding, consider suppositories medicated with cortisone.	
Insomnia	1. Anxiety. 2. Discomforts of late pregnancy. 3. Normal changes in the sleep/wake cycle in late pregnancy. 4. Early labor.	1. Depression. 2. Anxiety, worry. 3. Stress.	General measures: 1. Alleviate or reduce sources of anxiety. 2. Avoid stimulation activity just before bedtime. 3. Read a dull book. 4. Take a hot bath. 5. Use massage techniques. 6. Use relaxation techniques. 7. Drink hot liquids such as herb teas, Unisom 20 mg, or L-tryptophan, 500–1000 mg before retiring.	History of or present depression, anxiety, difficulty with concentration, anorexia, anemia, exercise intolerance, chest pain or discomfort.

			8. Exercise regularly during day. 9. Modify schedule to allow for naps during day. 10. Avoid regular use of alcohol & sleeping pills. 11. Deal with specific concern; refer if necessary to mental health counselor. 12. Alleviate specific discomforts of pregnancy where possible. 13. Conserve energy at beginning of labor.	
Leg cramps	Not clear. Theories include: 1. Inadequate or impaired calcium intake. 2. Lack of balance in the calcium/phosphorus ratio in the body. 3. Pressure from the enlarging uterus on the nerves to the lower extremities. Occur primarily in second and third trimesters.	1. Varicosities. 2. Thrombophlebitis. 3. Excessive activity (especially prolonged standing or walking in high heels). 4. Dehydration. 5. Nerve root compression.	Comfort measures: 1. Straighten affected leg and point heel. 2. General exercise and a habit of good body mechanics to improve circulation. 3. Elevate leg periodically throughout day. 4. Diet review: balance calcium and phosphorus intake. Calcium: diary products, calcium gluconate or lactate, or Tums. Phosphorus: foods rich in protein. Watch for excess phosphorus (excessive protein or soda).	History of deep-vein thromboembolytic disease, presence of Homans's sign, abnormal pulses in one or both lower extremities, redness, tenderness, heat, swelling, coldness, numbness, or whiteness in calf or leg.

(*continued*)

(Continued)

Discomfort	Etiology	Differential Diagnosis	Relief Measures	Danger Signs
Leukorrhea	High levels of estrogen cause increased vascularity & hypertrophy of cervical glands and vaginal cells, so production increases.	1. Ruptured membranes. 2. Vaginitis. 3. Cervicitis. 4. Condyloma acuminatum 5. Genital herpes. 6. STDs & cervical dysplasias or neoplasia.	1. Keep vulva clean & dry. 2. Avoid pantyhose & tight or layered clothing. 3. Wear cotton underwear or a nightgown without underwear at night. 4. If using pantyliners, use unscented/nondeodorant ones & change frequently. 5. Avoid douching & tampon use. 6. Avoid large amounts of simple sugars & add lactobacillus. 7. Eat sugar-free, active culture yogurt if taking antibiotics.	Green, watery, bloody, itchy, or irritating discharge that smells foul or fishy, fever, flu-like symptoms, abdominal pain, bleeding after intercourse, dyspareunia, Candida, trichomonads, clue cells & abnormal numbers of coccal, bacteria, red and white blood cells are present microscopically.
Nausea	Unknown etiology, theories include: 1. Sudden rise in hormone levels, especially estrogen. 2. Endocrine effect on the CNS center that controls N & V.	1. Severe emotional problems. 2. Hyperemesis gravidarum. 3. Hydatidiform mole. 4. Hiatal hernia. 5. Gastroenteritis.	1. Maintain high carbohydrate diet. 2. Avoid spicy, greasy food and those with strong or offensive odors. 3. Eat small, frequent meals. 4. Avoid large amounts of fluids at one time, with meals. 5. Keep crackers, popcorn, or dry toast at bedside to eat before arising.	Fever; lethargy; muscle aches; abdominal pain; cramping; diarrhea; jaundice; dark urine. Changes in shape or color of bowel movements, vaginal bleeding, head injury, HA.

3. Smooth muscle relaxation of the stomach & intestine, caused by increased progesterone levels.	6. Multiple gestation.	6. Eat or drink something sweet before going to bed and before getting up (peppermint tea, hot lemonade, or lemon juice, hard lemon candy).
4. Decrease in muscular peristalsis, tone, & secretion of acid & pepsin.	7. Cholecystitis.	7. Do not permit stomach to get completely empty—eat every 2–3 hr, immediately on awakening and before retiring, and in middle of night if awake.
	8. Hepatitis.	
	9. Inner ear infection.	
5. Overeating.	10. Sinusitis.	
6. Enlarging uterus in last half of pregnancy.	11. Diabetes.	8. Drink 1/4–1/2 cup. grapefruit juice with meals to increase stomach acidity.
	12. Thyroid dysfunction.	
7. Emotional factors.	13. Increased intracranial pressure.	9. Vitamin B_6 50–100 mg twice a day.
	14. Migraine HA.	10. May try Unisom 10 mg in morning and 1 tablet at night with vitamin B_6.
	15. Pica.	
	16. Food poisoning.	11. Ginger root 800–1000 mg twice a day and PRN.
		12. May take antiemetic medication (Tigan, Phenergan, or Compazine) is prescribed.
		13. Refer to dietician.
		14. May need hospitalization if significant dehydration, weight loss, or persistent ketonuria.

projectile vomiting, vomiting blood, neurologic signs, ataxia, chest pain ear pain, dehydration, or psychosocial distress.

(continued)

(Continued)

Discomfort	Etiology	Differential Diagnosis	Relief Measures	Danger Signs
Nocturia	1. Enlargement of uterus in pelvis causing pressure on bladder during first trimester. 2. Third trimester: a. pressure from fetal presenting parts; b. hyperplasia & hyperemia of pelvic organs; and c. increased kidney output.	1. UTI. 2. Pyelonephritis. 3. Gestational diabetes. 4. Pre-existing diabetes mellitus. 5. Hypocalcemia. 6. Spontaneous rupture of membranes.	1. Rest & sleep in lateral recumbent position to encourage kidney function. 2. Perform Kegel exercises. 3. Maintain adequate fluid intake (6–8 glasses of water). 4. Decrease water intake 2–3 hr before bedtime. 5. Discontinue drinking beverages that contain caffeine.	Back pain; fever; flu-like symptoms; hematuria; dysuria; urgency; dribbling; suprapubic pain; positive nitrazine or fern test, CVAT.
Round ligament pain	These are supporting structures for the uterus, and as uterus grows in pregnancy, the ligaments become stretched and often contract, resulting in sharp pain along the side of the abdomen, just above the groin area, usually	1. PID. 2. Appendicitis. 3. Gallbladder disease. 4. Peptic ulcer. 5. Pancreatitis. 6. Other GI or abdominal disease. 7. UTI. 8. Placental abruption.	1. Physician can explain reason for pain & reassure. 2. Comfort measures: a. avoid sudden movement; b. apply heat; c. try a change of activity; d. maternity girdle may be helpful; e. support uterus with a pillow when sitting or lying down; f. may take Tylenol 650 mg every 4 hr PRN. 3. If no relief, refer to physical therapist.	Contractions; constipation; diarrhea; low-grade fever; anorexia; periumbilical or right lower abdominal flank pain or tenderness; tender lump in groin that worsens with standing; one-sided constant pain

Shortness of Breath 61

	accentuated by sudden movements, coughing, lifting, etc.	9. Labor.	4. Call if sharp abdominal pain does not subside within 30 min.	that increases (if pregnancy is <14–16 wk); cervical dilatation, effacement or softening; rupture of membranes; adnexal or abdominal masses; hernias; decreased bowel sounds.
Shortness of breath	1. Enlarging uterus presses against abdominal organs & diaphragm, preventing full expansion of lungs. 2. Increased awareness of need to breathe. 3. May be aggravated by pressure of gravid uterus against vena cava, reducing venous return to heart.	1. URI. 2. Pulmonary or cardiac problems.	1. Avoid exercise that precipitates dyspnea & rest after exercise. 2. Avoid restrictive clothing. 3. Sitting up very straight, elevating head with pillows, or lying in lateral recumbent position may help.	HA; sore throat; coughing; flu-like symptoms; chest pain; indigestion; exercise intolerance with vomiting, sweating, or anxiety; history of smoking, respiratory, or cardiac problems.

(*continued*)

Part II: Common Discomforts of Pregnancy

(Continued)

Discomfort	Etiology	Differential Diagnosis	Relief Measures	Danger Signs
Supine hypotensive syndrome	Pooling of blood in lower extremities, expansion of vena cava & compression of the vena cava & lungs by the uterus.	1. Orthostatic hypotension. 2. Compression of the vena cava. 3. Hyperventilation. 4. Anemia. 5. Substance abuse. 6. Exposure to toxic agent. 7. Psychosocial stress. 8. CNS, cardiac, respiratory, endocrine, eye, ear, or sinus pathology.	1. Rest in lateral recumbent position. 2. Change position gradually, holding on to something when rising, or lower head below level of heart if feeling faint. 3. Apply compression stockings before getting out of bed & perform leg pumping exercises.	History of exposure to toxic agents; reports of substance abuse, sinus, or ear problems; numbness or tingling in digits or around mouth; nausea or vomiting; melena; heart palpitations; shortness of breath; double vision; loss of strength or sensation; incoordination; anxiety, depression; anemia.
Tingling & numbness of fingers	Increased lordosis & pressure on lower back with thrust of shoulders forward. Most common and night & early in the morning. May progress to partial anesthesia and impairment of manual proprioception.	1. Carpal tunnel syndrome. 2. Brachialgia. 3. Herniated intervertebral (cervical disk). 4. Hyperventilation.	1. Practice good posture. 2. Elevate affected hand. 3. Sleep with hand(s) elevated on pillows. 4. Perform stretching & relaxation exercises for shoulders. 5. Perform exercises to strengthen shoulder muscles. 6. Use splinting. 7. When hyperventilating, breathe into paper bag or cupped hands.	Paresthesia over thumb, index &/or middle fingers, & medial portion of the ring finger; pain in lateral aspect of hand & forearm; blanching of fingers; pain, loss of sensation &/or numbness in hand, wrist, or arm.

| Varicosities | 1. Familial tendency.
2. Impaired venous circulation & increased venous pressure in the extremities due to pressure of enlarging uterus.
3. Increased levels of progesterone causes relaxation of the vein walls and valves and surrounding smooth muscle.
4. Constrictive clothing or prolonged periods of standing, which impairs venous return from the extremities. | 1. Venous thrombosis.
2. Thrombophlebitis.
3. Edema from PIH.
4. Physiologic edema of pregnancy. | Preventive measures:
1. Avoid constrictive clothing, long periods of standing and sitting, crossing legs when sitting.
2. Whenever possible, sit (with legs elevated) rather than stand.
3. Maintain good posture, and good body mechanics.
Treatment measures:
1. Wear support hose.
2. Take rest periods through day.
3. Lie on back with legs straight and at a 45° angle for 20 min several times daily.
4. For vulvar varicosities: lie on shoulders, with body and legs straight from the waist and at 45° angle to waist (resting against wall) for 15–20 min several times a day; support vulva with foam rubber pad or perineal pad held in place with sanitary belt; lie on side or back with hips elevated for 15–20 min several times daily. | History of or present clotting, swelling, redness, or tenderness; cold, white, numb leg; inflammation over varicosities; dependent cyanosis; presence of Homans's sign; deep pain on palpation; distention of veins on dorsal side of foot after elevation; presence of Louvel's sign; restlessness; fever; tachycardia. |

III

Management of Common Problems and Procedures

ABRUPTIO PLACENTA

I. **Definition:** Premature separation of the normally implanted placenta at any time before delivery of the baby. Varies from small area to complete separation. Types are:
   A. Marginal sinus: A small margin of the placenta separates.
   B. Mild: Includes marginal, very small area separated.
   C. Moderate: At least one fourth but less than two thirds separated.
   D. Severe: More than two thirds of the placenta is separated.

II. **Etiology**
   A. Incidence is about 1 in 150 births
   B. More frequent in multiparas
   C. More frequent in women over age 35
   D. More frequent if hypertension is present
   E. Trauma to the abdomen may contribute
      1. Direct blow to the uterus
      2. Forceful external version
      3. Needle puncture at amniocentesis
   F. Rapid reduction of uterine size and pressure after rupture of membranes in polyhydramnios
   G. Malnutrition
   H. Short umbilical cord
   I. Smoking

III. **Clinical Features:** see Table 3-1.

IV. **Complications**
   A. Hemorrhage and resulting shock
   B. Hemorrhage may shear off remaining attached placenta.
   C. Force of collecting blood in uterus may cause:
      1. Rupture into amniotic sac
      2. Extravasation between muscle fibers of the myometrium (Couvelaire's uterus) causes irritable uterus and inability to relax its tone.
   D. Disseminated intravascular coagulation—due to myometrial damage and large amount of blood clotting
   E. Renal disturbances secondary to shock and/or clotting disturbances
   F. Fetal distress due to hemorrhaging
   G. Renal failure secondary to ischemia
   H. Pituitary necrosis (Sheehan's syndrome) secondary to ischemia
   I. Hepatitis secondary to massive blood transfusions

V. **Management**
   A. Consult with physician immediately for *all* cases.
   B. Rh(D) negative patients: All unsensitized Rh(D) negative patients should receive a RhoGAM injection after each uterine bleeding episode to prevent sensitization from possible mixing of Rh(D)

Table 3-1. Clinical Features of Abruptio Placenta

Symptoms	Mild	Moderate	Severe
Bleeding	Dark, none to moderate	Scant to moderate, may be up to 1000 ml behind placenta	Moderate to profuse
Fetus	No distress	Distress	Severe distress, dead
Uterine Tone	Poor uterine relaxation between contractions	Little relaxation between contractions	Extreme rigidity
Pain	None or vague lower abdomen discomfort	Tender	Agonizing, tearing, knifelike, un-remitting
Shock	None	Varies	Severe
Psychological	No change noted	Vague to moderate anxiety	Extremely anxious
Other	Uterine irritability noted	Fetal heart tone hard to hear with external monitor	Fetal heart tones may be absent; Uterine size increases as it fills with blood

positive fetal blood with maternal blood. The usual dose is 1 vial, which is adequate for a transfusion of up to 15 ml of fetal blood into the maternal circulation. The dosage should be larger if it is possible that more than 15 ml was transfused. A Kleinhauer-Betke test can be ordered to determine the amount of fetal blood in the maternal circulation.

AMENORRHEA

I. **Definition**
   A. Primary
      1. No period by age 14 in the presence of normal growth and development of secondary sexual characteristics. Menses usually begins within 12 months after the appearance of pubic hair.
      2. No period by age 16, regardless of the presence of normal growth and development, and appearance of secondary sexual characteristics.
   B. Secondary: Absence of periods for over 6 months in a woman who has established her menstrual cycle.

II. **Etiology**
   A. Primary amenorrhea
      1. Abnormal chromosomes
      2. Anatomic defects
         a. Imperforate hymen
         b. Vaginal agenesis
      3. Emotional stress
      4. Excessive exercise
      5. Bulimia/anorexia
   B. Secondary amenorrhea
      1. Pregnancy
      2. Menopause
      3. Pituitary disorder
      4. Obesity
      5. Eating disorders
      6. Excessive exercise
      7. Rapid weight loss
      8. Cessation of menses following use of oral contraception or Depo-Provera
      9. Stress
      10. Thyroid disease
      11. Polycystic ovary disease
      12. Some medications

III. **Clinical Features**
   A. History
      1. Menstrual history
      2. Contraceptive history
      3. Sexual history
      4. Symptoms of galactorrhea
      5. Family history of sexual development

6. Medications
7. Sources of emotional stress
8. Symptoms of climacteric
9. History of chronic illness
10. Present weight, weight 1 year ago
B. Physical exam
 1. Neck: thyroid gland—enlarged?
 2. Heart: rhythm/rate, palpitations?
 3. Breasts: check for:
   a. Development
   b. Discharge (milky/clear, dark/light, thick/thin)
 4. Vaginal exam: check for:
   a. Imperforate hymen
   b. Atrophic vagina
   c. Absence of cervical mucous
 5. Bimanual exam: check for:
   a. Enlarged uterus
   b. Enlarged, cystic ovaries

VI. **Laboratory**
A. Primary—perform chromosomal karyotyping
B. Human chorionic gonadotropin (hCG)
C. Prolactin level
D. Thyroid-stimulating hormone
E. Follicle-stimulating hormone
F. Luteinizing hormone
G. Dehydroepiandrosterone sulfate
H. Sequential Multiple Analyzer Computer (SMAC)/complete blood count (CBC) for suspected eating disorder
I. Serum testosterone if patient is hirsute
J. Papanicolaou (Pap) smear

VII. **Management**
A. If hCG is positive, patient is pregnant.
B. If hCG is negative, give 5 to 10 mg medroxyprogesterone acetate (Provera) orally for 5 to 10 days or progesterone in oil 100 to 200 mg IM.
 1. If no withdrawal bleeding, give 1 to 2 mg of Estrace or 0.625 to 2.5 mg of Premarin orally for 25 days. Give 5 to 10 mg of Provera orally days 16 to 25 of cycle. If no bleeding, repeat one time.
 2. If withdrawal bleeding with Provera, the patient is anovulatory and should be instructed to call if no menses within 90 days. (To protect against unopposed estrogen effects, a period is necessary every 3 to 4 months.)

a. If sexually active, an hCG test must be done before each cycle of Provera.
   b. Consider oral contraceptives.
C. If breast discharge present, do work up (see Galactorrhea guidelines on page 132).
D. If thyroid-stimulating hormone is elevated, diagnosis is primary hypothyroidism; refer as appropriate.
E. If prolactin level is above 20 mg/ml and all other tests are negative, give Parlodel 2.5 mg every day; if above 80 mg/ml, request magnetic resonance imaging or coned down view of sella turcica. The patient may have a pituitary tumor.
   1. If abnormal, refer for further studies.
   2. If normal sella turcica, give Parlodel to reduce prolactin to normal level. If prolactin level remains above 30 mg/ml after 2 months, obtain consultation.
F. Elevated follicle-stimulating hormone: diagnosis is ovarian failure. Is the patient menopausal?

NOTES

ANEMIA

I. **Definition:** Hemoglobin (Hgb) less than 12 in nonpregnant women or less than 10 in pregnant women.[1]
II. **Etiology**
   A. Acquired
      1. Iron deficiency anemia
      2. Anemia from blood loss
      3. Megaloblastic anemia
      4. Acquired hemolytic anemia
      5. Pernicious anemia
   B. Hereditary
      1. Thalassemia
      2. Sickle cell anemia
      3. Hereditary hemolytic anemia
III. **Clinical Features**
   A. History
      1. Heavy menses
      2. Chronic blood loss
      3. Family history
      4. Poor diet
      5. Closely spaced pregnancies
      6. Anemia with previous pregnancies
      7. Pica
   B. Signs and symptoms
      1. Fatigue, malaise, drowsiness
      2. Dizziness, weakness
      3. Headaches
      4. Sore tongue and mouth
      5. Anorexia, nausea, vomiting
      6. Skin pallor
      7. Pale mucous membranes, conjunctiva
      8. Pale fingernail beds
      9. Tachycardia
IV. **Management**
   A. At initial visit
      1. History of anemia, blood clotting problems, sickle cell disease, G6PD, or other hereditary hemolytic disease

---

[1]Cunningham FG, MacDonald P, Grant N, Leveno K, Gilstrap L. 1993.

2. Family history
B. Order CBC at initial visit
   1. Morphology
      a. Normal morphology indicates mature healthy red blood cells (RBCs).
      b. Microcytic, hypochromic RBCs indicate iron deficiency anemia.
      c. Macrocytic, hypochromic RBCs indicate pernicious anemia.
   2. Hemoglobin and hematocrit in pregnancy
      a. Hbg greater than 13, hematocrit (Hct) greater than 40: may indicate hypovolemia. Be alert for dehydration, pre-eclampsia.
      b. Hgb 11.5 to 13, Hct 34 to 40: normal, healthy
      c. Hgb 10.5 to 11.5, Hct 31 to 32: low normal. Recommend one to two iron tablets per day in addition to prenatal vitamin containing iron.
      d. Hgb 10, Hct 30: Anemic
         (1) Diet counsel, refer to dietitian, or both.
         (2) Supplemental iron two to three tablets a day or 1 time-release capsule, such as Slow Fe every day
      e. Hgb 9 to 10, Hct 27 to 30: Suspect megaloblastic anemia.
         (1) Diet counsel and refer to dietitian.
         (2) Chromagen twice a day, Ferro folic 500 mg twice a day, Niferex, 150 forte every day
      f. Hgb less than 9, Hct less than 27, or anemia that does not respond to above treatment measures:
         (1) Look for occult bleeding, infection.
         (2) The following labwork may be ordered:
            (a) Hgb and Hct (to rule out lab error)
            (b) Serum iron concentration level
            (c) Iron-binding capacity
            (d) Cell indices (white blood cell [WBC]; RBC counts)
            (e) Reticulocyte count (measures the production of erythrocytes)
            (f) Platelet count
            (g) Stool guaiac for occult bleeding
            (h) Stool culture for ova and parasites
            (i) G6PD screen (see Guidelines on page 75) if client is African American.
         (4) Consult with physician.
         (5) Diet counsel and refer to dietitian.
C. Check Hct at initial visit, 28 weeks, and 4 weeks after initiating therapy.
   1. Manage signs of anemia (according to section IV. B-2).

2. Consult with physician if:
   a. There is a steadily downward trend in Hct despite treatment.
   b. There is a significant drop in Hct over previous readings (rule out lab error first).
   c. There is no response to treatment after 4 to 6 weeks.
   d. At any time Hgb is below 9.0 or Hct is equal to or below 27%.

NOTES

ANEMIA: ACQUIRED HEMOLYTIC

I. **Definition:** An inherited, X-linked enzymatic defect in which the body does not produce the G6PD enzyme, which acts as a catalyst for aerobic use of glucose by RBCs. Seen in African Americans, Asians, and persons of Mediterranean descent.

II. **Etiology**
   A. Two percent of all African American women have the disease.
   B. Infections and several oxident drugs in the presence of G6PD deficiency will precipitate RBC hemolysis with resultant mild-to-severe hemolytic anemia.

III. **Management**
   A. Screening: Patients who are African American who have anemia or frequent urinary tract infections (UTIs) should have a G6PD screen.
   B. Treatment
      1. Prescribe 1 mg folic acid every day.
      2. Give patient a list of medicines to avoid.
      3. If pregnant, obtain urine culture and sensitivity (C&S) monthly.
      4. Consult with physician when in crisis, severe anemia.
   C. Medications to avoid
      1. Aldomet
      2. Antimalarial drugs
      3. Aspirin
      4. Ascorbic acid (massive doses)
      5. Chloramphenicol
      6. Co-trimoxide (Bactrim, Septra)
      7. Diaphenylsulfone
      8. Isoniazid
      9. Methylene blue
      10. N^1-Acetylsufanilamide
      11. Nalidixic acid
      12. Naphthalene (moth balls)
      13. Nitrofurantoin
      14. Nitrofurazone
      15. Orinase
      16. Para-aminosalicylic acid
      17. Pentaquine
      18. Phenacetin
      19. Primaquine
      20. Probenecid
      21. Quinacrine (atabrine)
      22. Quinidine

23. Quinine
24. Quinocide
25. Sulfasalazine (Azulfidine)
26. Sulfa
27. Sulfacetamide
28. Sulfamethoxypyridazine (Kynex)
29. Sulfanilamide
30. Sulfapyridine
31. Sulfisoxazole (Gantrisin)
32. Sulfoxone

NOTES

ANEMIA: IRON DEFICIENCY

I. **Definition and Etiology**
   A. Characteristics
      1. Most common anemia of pregnancy: constitutes about 95% of pregnancy-related anemias.
      2. Morphology: RBCs microcytic, hypochromic
      3. Serum iron is decreased, iron-binding capacity is increased.

II. **Clinical Features**
   A. Suspect if:
      1. One or more of the predisposing factors for anemia exist.
      2. Hct less than 32
   B. Diagnosis confirmed if:
      1. Morphology: microcytic, hypochromic RBCs
      2. Serum iron saturation: less than 15% after the patient is off iron therapy for 1 week.

III. **Management**
   A. Routine screening
      1. At the initial visit, ask about any past history of anemia or blood clotting problems.
      2. Order CBC at initial visit.
      3. Discuss the importance of taking prenatal vitamins (with iron).
      4. Recheck Hct at 28 weeks of pregnancy.
   B. Treatment of anemia
      1. Hgb less than 11, Hct less than 34%:
         a. Diet counsel.
            (1) Review patient's diet.
            (2) Discuss dietary sources of iron.
            (3) Give handout on foods high in iron.
            (4) Offer referral to dietitian.
         b. Advise supplemental iron in addition to prenatal vitamin. Iron requirement in pregnancy is 60 mg elemental iron.
            (1) Time-released iron tablets are best but much more expensive. Any standard iron salt preparation is adequate.
            (2) Take one to three tablets daily in divided doses.
            (3) Iron is better absorbed on an empty stomach. Take 1 hour before meals or 2 hours after meals.
            (4) Vitamin C aids iron absorption. Take iron with a juice high in vitamin C or a vitamin C tablet.
            (5) Antacids and dairy products can hinder absorption.
            (6) It is preferable to take iron with antacids or food than not to take it at all.

2. If Hgb less than 10, Hct less than 30%, consider megaloblastic anemia (see Guidelines on page 79).
3. If Hgb less than 9, Hct less than 28%, manage according to Anemia Guidelines.
4. If Hgb less than 9, Hct less than or equal to 27%, at start of labor:
   a. Patient should be comanaged with physician.
   b. Consider intravenous (IV) or heparin lock in labor.

NOTES

ANEMIA: MEGALOBLASTIC

I. **Definition and Etiology**
   A. An anemia in which the RBCs are reduced in number and are macrocytic and hypochromic
   B. Commonly associated with iron-deficiency anemia. It's rare to see megaloblastic anemia alone.
   C. Associated with a diet lacking in fresh vegetables and/or animal protein

II. **Clinical Features**
   A. Symptoms
      1. Nausea, vomiting
      2. Anorexia
   B. Morphology
      1. Hypochromic, macrocytic RBCs
      2. A low Hgb/Hct that does not respond to iron therapy
      3. Diet history indicating low intake of fresh vegetables, animal protein, or both

III. **Management**
   A. Supplements
      1. Prenatal vitamin containing folic acid and iron
      2. Folic acid 1 to 2 mg per day to correct folic acid deficiency.
      3. Supplemental iron, since megaloblastic anemia rarely exists in the absence of iron-deficiency anemia.
   B. Diet counsel.
      1. Review patient's diet.
      2. Advise dietary sources of folic acid.
      3. Offer referral to dietitian.
   C. CBC
      1. Repeat CBC in 1 month.
      2. Should notice an increase in the reticulocyte count of 3% to 4% in 2 to 3 weeks, and a slight increase in the Hgb/Hct count.
      3. If no response, consult physician.

ANEMIA: PERNICIOUS

I. **Definition and Etiology**
   A. Pernicious anemia is caused by lack of intrinsic factor in the gastric juices, which is necessary for the absorption of vitamin B_{12} from food. Because B_{12} is not absorbed, the RBCs do not mature normally.
   B. It is rarely seen in persons under age 35

II. **Clinical Features**
   A. Macrocytic RBCs, which may also be normochromic or hyperchromic
   B. RBCs may easily be mistaken for those seen in folic acid deficiency.
   C. Treatment with folic acid may mask pernicious anemia because the RBCs may become normocytic even though the disease still exists.

III. **Diagnosis**
   A. Suspect pernicious anemia if, after treatment with folic acid, the RBCs become normal in morphology but the hematocrit does not increase.
   B. Diagnosis may be made if improvement occurs after a trial treatment with parenteral B_{12} 1000 ng for 3 months.

IV. **Management**
   A. Review patient's diet for animal products. If diet is lacking in sources of vitamin B_{12}, give diet counseling.
   B. Parenteral B_{12} 1 cc (1000 nanograms) IM every month
   C. Offer referral to dietitian.
   D. Repeat CBC in 1 month.
      1. Condition is alleviated if:
         a. Morphology is normal.
         b. Hematocrit is increased.
      2. If no change, consult with physician.

NOTES

ANEMIA: SICKLE CELL

I. **Definition and Etiology**
   A. Types
      1. In sickle cell trait, there is one normal gene and one Hgb-S gene. Symptoms do not appear except in severe oxygen deprivation.
      2. In sickle cell disease, both genes are Hbg-S. The disease is chronic and debilitating. Morbidity and mortality are high.
   B. Incidence
      1. One in 12 African Americans has sickle cell trait.
      2. One in 500 African Americans has the disease.

II. **Management**
   A. Order a sickle cell screen on all African American patients
      1. If negative, both genes are normal and no problem exists.
      2. If positive, order a hemoglobin electrophoresis.
         a. If homozygous, patient is considered high-risk and is referred to physician.
         b. If heterozygous, patient is considered low-risk, and can be managed normally throughout pregnancy and labor.
   B. Consider monthly urine C&S because of the increased risk of UTIs during pregnancy.
   C. Counseling
      1. Inform patient of her sickle cell trait.
      2. Advise testing of the father of the baby. If he is also heterozygous, there is a chance that the baby could have the disease.
      3. Refer for genetic counseling as necessary.

NOTES

BACKACHE

I. **Etiology**
   A. Softening of the pelvic ligaments during pregnancy
   B. Increasing weight of the uterus changes the woman's center of gravity, causing postural changes, which result in increased lumbar lordosis.
   C. Back strain due to:
      1. Excessive bending
      2. Excessive walking
      3. Improper lifting
   D. Lax abdominal muscle tone, especially in multiparas.

II. **Management**
   A. Use good body mechanics when reaching for something on the floor or lifting: bend the knees, keep the back straight rather than bending from the waist.
   B. Good posture when sitting or standing; avoid exaggerated lordosis.
   C. Avoid excessive bending, lifting, or walking without rest periods.
   D. Pelvic rock exercises to strengthen the lower back and relieve tension.
   E. Use flexion and stretch exercises to strengthen muscles.
   F. Wear supportive low-heeled shoes; avoid high-heeled shoes, which further exaggerate the lordosis.
   G. For sleeping
      1. Use a firm mattress.
      2. Use pillows for support, to straighten out the back, and alleviate pulling and strain on the back.
   H. If the problem is due to lax abdominal muscles, a maternity girdle may help.
   I. Heat to the area.
   J. Tylenol orally every 4 hours needed for minor discomfort.
   K. Offer referral to physician if:
      1. The problem persists despite above measures
      2. Persistent muscle spasm
      3. Severe or significant hindrance to activities of daily living

III. **Differential Diagnosis**
   A. Rule out UTI (see Guidelines on page 244). If any question, get urine C&S.
   B. Rule out labor. Question regarding timing of backache (eg, rhythmicity, associated with uterine hardening). If any question, assess with external fetal monitor, ascertain if cervical changes occur over time.

BACTERIAL VAGINOSIS

I. **Definition:** A sexually transmitted vaginal infection caused by the Gardnerella bacteria, which is aerobic.

II. **Etiology**
   A. The second most common cause of vaginitis after Monilia.
   B. Does not invade the vaginal mucosa; tissue underlying the discharge is healthy.
   C. A significant percentage of women are asymptomatic.
   D. Although not usually symptomatic in males, they can harbor it in their urethra and transmit it to the woman.
   E. Implicated in chorioamnionitis, premature delivery

III. **Clinical Features**
   A. Signs and symptoms
      1. May be asymptomatic.
      2. Major presenting symptom is yellow or creamy-gray vaginal discharge and a fishy odor.
      3. Vaginal mucosa may look normal.
      4. Usually not associated with pain, burning, or itching.
      5. If present, look for a concomitant infection.
   B. Laboratory findings
      1. Positive sniff test when mixed with potassium hydroxide.
      2. Microscopic findings on wet mount: Clue cells (epithelial cells, which appear "sandy" because they are studded with the Gardnerella bacteria).

IV. **Management**
   A. Make diagnosis. (See Vaginal Discharge Guidelines on page 249 for differential diagnosis.)
   B. Considerations regarding treatment:
      1. Flagyl (metronidazole) orally or vaginally is the drug of choice. If unable to take, ampicillin 500 mg orally four times a day for 7 days can be given.
      2. Treatment of the male partner is controversial. It seems prudent to evaluate or treat steady partners. Condoms should be used until 1 week after treatment is completed.
   C. Treatment in first trimester of pregnancy
      1. It is acceptable to avoid treatment in first trimester.
         a. Gardnerella is often asymptomatic and not associated with any particular ill effects in pregnancy.
         b. Most treatment measures have variable effectiveness and are often found to be less than satisfactory.
         c. Metronidazole, the most effective treatment measure, is contraindicated in first trimester.

2. If symptomatic, try one of the following:
    a. MetroGel Vaginal cream 1 application every day or twice a day for 5 to 7 days.
    b. Ampicillin 500 mg orally four times a day for 7 days
    c. Terazol, Femstat, AVC, Tri-Sulfa, or other vaginal creams/suppositories
D. If present in second or third trimester, effective treatment is desirable because of the association between Gardnerella, premature rupture of membranes, and postpartum endometritis. Use one of the following:
    1. Metronidazole 250 to 500 mg orally twice to three times a day for 5 to 7 days.
    2. MetroGel Vaginal cream, one applicator vaginally at bedtime for 5 to 7 days.
    3. Ampicillin 500 mg tablets orally four times a day for 7 days.
E. With treatment by either metronidazole or penicillin, warn patient that Monilia vaginitis may develop secondary to antibiotic therapy. She should be alert for signs and symptoms and may want to use prophylactic vaginal yogurt, or acidophilus tablets, as well as pharmaceuticals while taking antibiotics.

NOTES

BLEEDING IN PREGNANCY UNDER 20 WEEKS' GESTATION

I. **Definition and Etiology:** Approximately 20% of pregnant women experience vaginal bleeding during the first trimester. Less than half of these women will have a spontaneous abortion (SAB). Causes of bleeding under 20 weeks' gestation include:
   A. Implantation bleeding
   B. Threatened spontaneous abortion
   C. Inevitable spontaneous abortion
   D. Incomplete spontaneous abortion
   E. Complete spontaneous abortion
   F. Missed spontaneous abortion
   G. Ectopic pregnancy
   H. Gestational trophoblastic neoplasia (GTN)
   I. Cervicitis
   J. Cervical polyps
   K. Cervical carcinoma
   L. Normal hyperemia of the cervix
   M. Unknown etiology

II. **Clinical Features**
   A. Implantation bleeding
      1. Occurs 1 to 2 weeks after conception.
      2. It is caused by blood escaping from blood vessels in the uterine epithelium that have been eroded by the implanting fertilized ovum.
      3. Bleeding is usually scant, light pink, unaccompanied by pain, and lasts only 1 to 2 days.
   B. Threatened abortion
      1. Vaginal bleeding with or without pelvic cramping and backache during the first trimester
      2. No cervical changes observed.
      3. Approximately 50% of threatened SABs do progress to complete SABs.
   C. Inevitable spontaneous abortion
      1. Increase in vaginal bleeding, accompanied by increasingly severe pelvic cramping
      2. Evidence of cervical dilatation, and/or effacement with or without the presence of fetal membranes or placenta at the cervical os
      3. It is impossible to halt the progress of the SAB at this point.
   D. Incomplete spontaneous abortion
      1. Part of the products of conception remain within the uterine cavity, causing persistent, sometimes profuse, vaginal bleeding.
      2. Passage of tissue and clots, with a history of vaginal bleeding and cramping will persist until all the products of conception have been evacuated from the uterus.

E. Complete spontaneous abortion
   1. The uterus spontaneously evacuates itself of all the products of conception.
   2. Usually occurs before the 6th week or after the 14th week of pregnancy
F. Spontaneous missed abortion
   1. Products of conception are retained in the uterus after the embryo or fetus has died.
   2. May have previously had signs and symptoms of a threatened SAB, which appear to resolve except for occasional brown spotting.
   3. Eventually the symptoms of pregnancy disappear and the uterine size becomes smaller.
   4. The term "missed AB" is usually applied to retention of a dead embryo or fetus for at least 4 to 8 weeks.
G. Ectopic pregnancy (See Ectopic Pregnancy Guidelines on page 117.)
H. GTN or molar pregnancy
I. Cervicitis (See Chlamydia and Gonorrhea Guidelines on pages 96 and 137.)
J. Cervical polyps
   1. Painless bleeding, especially after coitus
   2. Bleeding appears early in gestation
   3. Appear as bright red pedunculated growths protruding from the cervical os
K. Cervical carcinoma
   1. Painless vaginal bleeding, often after coitus
   2. Cervical erosion often is seen on routine speculum exam
   3. Abnormal Pap smear results
L. Normal hyperemia of the cervix
   1. Spontaneous light vaginal spotting or bleeding, which may or may not be related to coitus
   2. Caused by the increased vascularization of the cervix that normally occurs during pregnancy

III. **Clinical Features**
   A. History
      1. Reports having, or having had, the symptoms of pregnancy
      2. Vaginal bleeding that can be scant, profuse; brown, pink, or bright red in color
      3. Abdominal pain, ranging from mild cramping to severe, sharp, unilateral pain
      4. Passage of tissue, blood clots, or grape-like vesicles (GTN)
      5. Bleeding that occurs at specific times (eg, postcoitally) or is unrelated to activity
      6. Exposure to and symptoms of STD

7. History of pelvic inflammatory disease (PID), previous ectopic pregnancy, intrauterine device (IUD) use, infertility, or adnexal surgery
8. Disappearance of subjective signs and symptoms of pregnancy (missed SAB)

B. Signs and symptoms
1. Uterine size
   a. Normal for dates in threatened SABs
   b. Size less than dates in incomplete and missed SABs and ectopic pregnancies
   c. Size will decrease in complete SABs.
   d. Size greater than dates in 50% of GTN cases
2. Cervical dilatation and effacement in inevitable SABs
3. Presence of products of conception at cervical os or in the vaginal vault in incomplete SABs
4. Nitrozine-positive fluid in vaginal vault in some cases of inevitable and incomplete SABs
5. Unilateral sausage-like enlargement of adnexa, usually accompanied by tenderness, is sometimes palpable in ectopic pregnancies
6. Bright red, pedunculated growth, protruding from the cervical os, may be observed if cervical polyp is causing the bleeding.
7. Cervical inflammation, erythema, friability, and leukorrhea may be seen in cervicitis.
8. Suspect SAB if absence of fetal heart tones (FHTs) with Doppler in a pregnancy over 12 weeks by size and dates; 14 weeks in obese patients

C. Diagnostic tests
1. Sonogram may indicate the presence or absence of a fetal sac, fetal heart pulsations, or "snowstorm" pattern (GTN). Fetal heart activity should be seen on a sonogram by 4 to 6 weeks of pregnancy.
2. CBC or hemoglobin and hematocrit (H&H), serial quantitative hCG type and Rh(D) if unknown
3. Cervical cultures for gonorrhea, chlamydia, and beta strep as necessary
4. Coagulation studies in patients with missed SABs due to the potential of disseminated intravascular coagulation developing. This is especially important if it has been 5 or more weeks since the death of the fetus, or 5 months after last menstrual period.

IV. Management
A. Threatened SAB
1. Bedrest until bleeding subsides
2. Pelvic rest for at least 2 weeks after the bleeding has stopped
3. Refrain from sexual intercourse.
4. If bleeding continues or is accompanied by the passage of clots or tissues, do an ultrasound and refer to a physician.

B. Inevitable, incomplete, complete, or missed abortion
   1. Ultrasound
   2. Quantitative beta human chorionic gonadotropin (QBHCG) (PRN)
   3. Refer to physician's care as indicated.
C. Ectopic pregnancy
   1. Ultrasound
   2. Consult with or refer to physician as soon as suspected.
D. If a patient with threatened SAB has resolution of her symptoms, continue routine prenatal care at 2-week intervals until normal uterine growth and FHTs are confirmed.
E. If anemia is present, then iron supplementation and high iron diet are prescribed. (See Anemia Guidelines on page 72.)
F. If patient is Rh(D) negative and she has a threatened SAB, incomplete or complete SAB, or ectopic pregnancy, she should have an injection of Rh(D) immune globulin (RhoGAM) or Rh(D) immune globulin micro-close if less than 12 weeks within 72 hours after the completion of the SAB or termination of ectopic pregnancy.
G. If cervical polyps are present, consultation/referral to physician for treatment is indicated. Or a trained practitioner if comfortable and the stock is visible, may remove the polyp and send to pathology.
H. Transfer to physician care all patients with vaginal bleeding during the first trimester when GTN is suspected or diagnosed.
I. Follow-up includes:
   1. If threatened SAB resolves, then patient is seen routinely.
   2. Appropriate documentation on problem list and progress notes.
   3. For patients who have aborted, contraception needs to be discussed. It is best to wait for two to three menstrual cycles before becoming pregnant again.

V. **Education**
   A. Discuss the diagnostic tests that will be ordered and interpretation of results.
   B. If a threatened SAB, inform the patient that she has a 50% chance of maintaining the pregnancy.
   C. Inform the patient that she should call if she develops a fever, has foul-smelling discharge, has profuse or prolonged bleeding, has passage of tissue or clots, or develops abdominal or low back pain. She should save any tissue passed.
   D. If an SAB has occurred, educate the patient regarding the normal course of recovery from a SAB, and the need to have follow-up evaluation of her physical and psychological status.
   E. If an SAB has occurred, help the patient and her partner to work through any guilt or grief regarding their loss. Refer as necessary.
   F. Give information on the administration of RhoGAM if patient is Rh(D) negative.

BLEEDING IN PREGNANCY OVER 20 WEEKS' GESTATION

I. **Etiology:** Vaginal bleeding in a pregnancy that is over 20 weeks' gestation can be due to:
   A. Abruptio placenta (see Guidelines on page 67)
      1. If bleeding is present, blood is usually dark, moderate in amount.
      2. Pain may range from vague to intense discomfort.
      3. Uterus increases in size as bleeding continues, ranges from mild irritability to extreme rigidity.
      4. Uterine tenderness may be absent, mild and localized, or marked and diffuse.
      5. FHT may be absent or difficult to auscultate.
   B. Placenta previa
      1. Painless hemorrhage
      2. Does not usually appear until near the end of the second trimester
      3. Blood usually bright red, may be slight to copious
      4. There is no uterine irritability, rigidity, or tenderness
   C. Cervical lesions
      1. Bleeding usually light
      2. History of vaginitis, cervicitis, polyps, condylomata, and so on
      3. Recent intercourse, which may cause spotting
   D. Bloody show
      1. Always a possibility at term
      2. Usually scant in amount, pinkish rather than bright red, and accompanied by mucous
   E. Uterine rupture
      1. Those at risk include:
         a. Women with a history of previous cesarean section or other uterine surgery
         b. Cephalopelvic disproportion (CPD) allowed to labor too long—the lower uterine segment continues to thin out as long as contractions continue and may rupture
         c. Improper use of oxytocin for induction or augmentation of labor; tetanic contractions may result in rupture
         d. Attempt at external or internal version
      2. The classic symptom is severe pain at time of a contraction, followed by sudden absence of pain and contractions.

III. **Management**
   A. History
      1. Type of bleeding
         a. Bright red—most likely with previa

        b. Dark brown—old blood, may be from earlier abruption or bloody show

        c. Serous—may indicate rupture of membranes

    2. Amount—if soaking more than two pads in an hour, needs immediate attention. Watch for shock.

    3. Weeks gestation

    4. Any pain? Most likely with abruption. Previa is characteristically painless.

B. Physical exam

    1. Assess color and amount of bleeding.

    2. Do not do manual vaginal exams until the cause of the bleeding is determined. An exam may rupture a placental vessel if there is a placenta previa, and cause instant severe hemorrhage. Use ultrasound.

    3. Assess vital signs, FHT, and signs of shock. Use external fetal monitor if bleeding significant.

    4. Order CBC, clot tube to hold, pro time, platelets, and fibrinogen if bleeding is excessive.

    5. Placenta previa and abruptio placenta can be diagnosed by ultrasound.

    6. If the patient is not in labor and placenta previa has been ruled out, a careful speculum exam may be done to assess the condition of the cervix. If cervical infection/lesions are present, treat according to guidelines.

C. Consult with physician if:

    1. Any frank bleeding

    2. There are signs of fetal compromise or maternal shock.

    3. The cause of the bleeding cannot be determined and/or treated by the nurse–midwife or practitioner.

D. If the situation is emergent:

    1. Summon physician immediately.

    2. Prepare for immediate caesarean section.

    3. Start IV of lactated Ringer's solution with large-bore intracath.

    4. Treat signs of shock (See Postpartum Hemorrhage Guidelines on page 200.).

    5. Keep flow sheet of vital signs, events, actions taken. Maintain continuous recording of FHT per monitor.

E. Treatment of the unsensitized Rh(D) negative patient

    1. Give RhoGAM injection after each uterine bleeding episode.

    2. Usual dose is 1 vial Rh(D) immune globulin, which is adequate for a transfusion of up to 15 ml of fetal blood into the maternal circulation.

    3. Dosage should be larger if it is possible that more than 15 ml was transfused.

    4. A Kleinhauer-Betke test can be ordered to determine the amount of fetal blood in the maternal circulation.

BREECH PRESENTATION

I. **Definition:** The presentation of the fetus in the uterus in which it is breech. The types are frank breech, complete breech, or footling breech.
II. **Etiology:** A breech presentation may be caused by some circumstance that prevents the normal version from taking place.
III. **Management**
   A. Before 30 to 32 weeks: Insignificant
   B. At 30 to 32 weeks: Incidence—14% of fetuses present breech
      1. Discuss with the patient the implication of breech presentation now and at term.
      2. Discuss danger signs.
      3. Be sure patient knows that she should inform care providers that the baby is breech.
      4. Instruct patient in doing breech turning exercises.
   C. At 36 weeks
      1. In most pregnancies, the fetus has assumed its final position by the 34th week.
      2. At term, only 3% to 4% of fetuses present in any position other than cephalic.
      3. Discuss pros and cons of vaginal breech delivery versus caesarean section.
      4. Refer to a physician to discuss options and make plans. An external version may be attempted at 37 weeks if primipara, and from 38 weeks to term in the multiparous patient. This needs to be done in the hospital, under ultrasound, with proper monitoring of patient and fetus.

NOTES

CARDIOVASCULAR ASSESSMENT

I. **Definition:** Evaluating the patient for physiologic changes and problems relating to the heart and blood vessels.

II. **Clinical Features:** Normal cardiovascular changes in pregnancy.
   A. Stroke volume increases by one third in the first 8 to 10 weeks.
      1. Increased estrogen levels cause the heart rate to increase 10 to 15 beats per minute in some women.
      2. Total blood volume increases by 20% to 30%.
         a. Plasma increases 40% to 50%.
         b. RBCs increase 20%.
   B. Reduction in exercise tolerance due to:
      1. Greater body weight to move around.
      2. Cardiac output already increased, less reserve for increase with exercise
   C. Progesterone causes blood vessel tone to decrease, so peripheral vascular resistance falls, leading to:
      1. Greater incidence of varicosities and aneurysms
      2. Drop in blood pressure (BP) at end of first trimester, returning to normal or slightly above in final weeks of pregnancy
   D. Diaphragm elevates and transverse diameter of thorax increases, pushing heart upward and to the left; it lies almost horizontally.
   E. Cardiac volume increases by about 75 ml.
   F. Systolic murmur may occur due to:
      1. Increased cardiac output
      2. Acceleration of blood flow (heart rate)
      3. Changes in position of heart
      4. Decreased blood viscosity—smaller ratio of RBCs to plasma
   G. Increased blood flow to most areas of the body from early pregnancy.

III. **Management: Cardiovascular Abnormalities**
   A. At the first visit, take a good history of the cardiovascular system.
      1. Any history of the following indicates consultation and workup by cardiologist:
         a. Palpitations, abnormalities in heart rate or rhythm.
         b. A nonproblematic (I/VI) murmur does not need a cardiac workup. Anything more than that requires referral to specialist.
         c. Any of the following, if chronic or of unknown cause:
            (1) Chest pain
            (2) Cyanosis
            (3) Dependent edema (differentiate from normal pregnancy edema)

2. Any history of the following indicates referral to an obstetrician for care:
   a. Rheumatic fever with resultant damage
   b. Heart disease or coronary artery disease
   c. Persistent hypertension
   d. Heart surgery
   e. Signs and symptoms of congestive heart failure
      (1) Persistent rales at base of lungs
      (2) Increased inability to carry out usual physical activity.
      (3) Increased dyspnea with exertion.
      (4) Hemoptysis
      (5) Cyanosis
      (6) Edema in lower extremities (differentiate from normal pregnancy edema)

B. Physical exam
   1. Routine assessment includes:
      a. Taking the BP
      b. Auscultating heart for:
         (1) Rate, rhythm, and quality of heart sounds at the four valvular areas
         (2) Extra sounds, murmurs, splitting, rubs, thrills
      c. Observation of the limbs for cyanosis, edema
   2. If the history or routine exam indicates possible abnormal cardiac function, perform a more extended exam.
      a. Observation of anterior chest wall for bulging, heaving, pulsation
      b. Palpation of anterior chest wall for point of maximum intensity (PMI), thrills, rubs
      c. Percussion of the anterior chest wall for heart size
   3. Consult with or refer to cardiologist for:
      a. Irregular heartbeat and/or tachycardia (over 100 beats per minute) in the absence of other findings indicative of heart disease or hyperthyroidism.
      b. Any systolic murmurs with a classification of greater than II/VI.

CERVICAL ABNORMALITIES

I. **Etiology**
   A. Congenital abnormalities/exposure to diethylstilbestrol (DES) in utero
   B. Atrophy/stenosis
   C. Cervicitis
   D. Endometriosis
   E. Erosion/ulcerations
   F. Human papilloma virus (HPV, condylomata)
   G. Polyps
   H. Trauma/surgery

II. **Clinical Features**
   A. Congenital abnormalities: Double cervix and other structural anomalies
   B. Atrophy/stenosis
      1. Menopausal women often have a pale cervix, small canal due to decreased estrogen.
      2. Cryosurgery, cone biopsy, postradiation
   C. Cervicitis
      1. Red, inflamed, friable
      2. Bleeds with intercourse
      3. Rule out chlamydia, neisseria gonorrhea, bacterial vaginosis, trichomonas, vaginitis, monilia, herpes.
   D. Endometriosis
      1. History suspicious of endometriosis or a diagnosis after laparoscopic exam
      2. Blue/black bump seen on cervix
   E. Erosion/ulcerations
      1. Rule out herpes
      2. History of tampax, cervical cap
   F. HPV
      1. May see warts on the cervix.
      2. Fifty to sixty percent of patients with external condylomata test positive on the cervix.
      3. Need to rule out herpes, nabothian cyst.
   G. Polyps
      1. History of spotting with intercourse
      2. Can sometimes see growth on stalk
   H. Trauma/surgery
      1. Trauma from delivery, elective abortion, instruments inserted into vagina
      2. LEEP, cone biopsy

III. **Management**
   A. Congenital abnormalities/exposure to DES in utero
      1. Congenital abnormalities may present problems in labor and delivery and need to be managed collaboratively with a physician.
      2. Exposure to DES in utero changes the location of the squamocolumnar junction, which is often located in the vagina rather than the ectocervix, predisposing the patient to more frequent cervical infections and cervical cancer. A Pap smear every year even when everything looks and has been normal is a must.
   B. Atrophy/stenosis
      1. Nothing further needed unless patient complains of vaginal dryness (see Menopause-HRT Guidelines on page 176).
   C. Cervicitis (See Guidelines on page 94.)
   D. Endometriosis—No management needed for cervical manifestation.
   E. Erosion/ulceration
      1. Treat cause.
      2. Amino Cerv at bedtime for 10 to 14 days
   F. HPV (See Guidelines on page 147.)
   G. Polyps
      1. May be removed if stalk can be seen
      2. Send to pathology.
   H. Trauma/surgery
      1. Monitor antepartal patients for an incompetent cervix.
      2. Cervix may fail to dilate or tear during labor.

NOTES

CHLAMYDIA

I. **Definition:** Infection by the organism *Chlamydia trachomatis*, a gram-negative intracellular parasite that is smaller than bacteria and larger than viruses.

II. **Incidence**
   A. Has been identified in half of men with nonspecific urethritis, and 20% to 60% of women with gonorrhea.
   B. The most prevalent STD in the United States today; several times more prevalent than gonorrhea.
   C. Five percent of babies born in the United States have a chlamydia infection; 50% of these develop conjunctivitis, and 20% develop pneumonia.

III. **Etiology**
   A. Often found in conjunction with other STDs
   B. The genus chlamydia has two species.
      1. *Chlamydia psittaci* is not an STD and not relevant in obstetric/gynecologic (OB/GYN) care. It is a mild flu-like disease, contracted following exposure to bird droppings containing the parasite.
      2. *Chlamydia trachomatis* is the STD species referred to in the remainder of this section and is responsible for the following diseases:
         a. Pelvic inflammatory disease
         b. Nongonococcal (and postgonococcal) urethritis
         c. Chronic conjunctivitis
            (1) May be sibling-associated where reinfection is generally more severe than the initial episode
            (2) Has been cited as a major cause of blindness
            (3) Adult infection is generally by exposure to genital discharges containing chlamydia.
         d. Chlamydiae blennorrhea:
            (1) Generally contracted by the fetus via passage through an infected birth canal
            (2) There are many clinical manifestations of this disease including:
               (a) Benign to severe conjunctivitis
               (b) Pneumonitis, which can become quite severe to fatal
         e. Lymphogranuloma venereum
            (1) A strain of *C. trachomatis* characterized by a transient minor genital ulcer and inguinal adenopathy (and possibly urethritis)
            (2) It can be cultured in the same specific medium as the other genital chlamydia, and is differentiated as the lymphogranuloma venereum strain on culture.

IV. **Clinical Features**
   A. Signs and symptoms (may be asymptomatic):
      1. Mucopurulent, foul-smelling vaginal discharge draining from the cervical os

2. Erythema, edema, congestion of cervix and vagina
3. Cervicitis
   a. Cobblestone ectopy
   b. Increased friability, bleeding
   c. Mucopurulent discharge from os
4. Urethritis
   a. Mild dysuria or lower abdominal pain
   b. Sterile pyuria
   c. Gradual onset
   d. Mucopurulent discharge from urethra

B. Conditions chlamydia can mimic
1. Cervicitis of chlamydia may look like cervicitis of herpes simplex. Chlamydia causes inflammation and ulceration of both ectocervix and endocervix, while herpes simplex affects ectocervix alone.
2. May result in a PID similar to that caused by gonorrhea.

C. May have a latency period of many decades, similar to syphilis, after initial infection.

D. Chlamydia is a major cause of:
1. Mucopurulent cervicitis
2. Urethral infection
3. PID and acute perihepatitis
4. Neonatal conjunctivitis and pneumonia

E. Chlamydiosis is associated with:
1. Infertility (secondary to PID)
2. Cervical dysplasia
3. Fetal wastage and stillbirth
4. Neonatal infections
5. Postpartum endometritis and salpingitis

V. **Management**

A. Suspect chlamydia in the following situations:
1. WBCs too numerous to count on a wet prep slide without large amounts of bacteria or yeast present.
2. Other STDs have been ruled out or treated unsuccessfully (especially in the presence of mucopurulent foul-smelling vaginal discharge, which is indicative of either gonorrhea or chlamydia).
3. Presence of dysuria and frequency, and UTI and urethritis have been ruled out.
4. Presence of cervicitis
5. Pap smear report is suggestive of chlamydia
6. Recent history of chlamydia, especially with symptoms
7. Partner has nongonococcal urethritis

B. All new OB patients and those suspected of, or exposed to, chlamydia need to be tested.
1. Specific tissue culture

a. Obtain chlamydia culture kit.
b. Swab transitional zone of cervix.
c. It is essential that enough epithelial cells be collected; swab area vigorously.
d. Cotton swabs are toxic to chlamydia. Use dacron swabs provided.
e. Results generally are obtained in 72 hours.
2. Rapid detection test for chlamydia antigen
a. Positive predictive value 100%, negative predictive value 94% to 98%.
b. May be done in the office. A cervical swab needs to be taken with the swabs provided with the kit.
c. Test results are ready within one-half hour.

C. Before beginning treatment, obtain Venereal Disease Research Laboratory (VDRL) test for syphilis and gonorrhea culture if not previously ruled out.
D. Treatment
1. Nonpregnant women not breastfeeding:
a. Zithromax (Z-Pak) taken on empty stomach; Zithromax oral suspension (Zithromax cocktail), which may be taken with food
b. Doxycycline 100 mg, 1 orally twice a day for 7 days
c. Ofloxacin 400 mg twice a day for 7 days
d. Amoxicillin 500 mg, 1 orally three times a day for 7 days
2. Pregnant or breastfeeding women:
a. Amoxicillin 500 mg, 1 orally three times a day for 7 days
b. Erythromycin 500 mg, 1 orally four times a day for 10 days; or erythromycin PCE (dispertab) 333 mg, 1 orally three times a day for 10 days
c. Zithromax (Z-Pak) taken on empty stomach; Zithromax oral suspension (Zithromax cocktail), which may be taken with food

E. Patient's partner(s) need to be referred for treatment. No sex while being treated to avoid reinfection. If unable to wait for test of cure (TOC), counsel to use condom.
F. Repeat cervical culture for TOC 6 weeks after treatment
1. If pregnant, re-examine cervix and repeat culture at 34 to 36 weeks' EGA
2. If culture is still positive, check:
a. Compliance with medications
b. If partner(s) received treatment
3. Repeat treatment with a different medication.

COLDS, FLU, UPPER RESPIRATORY INFECTION

I. **Etiology:** Usually viral; characterized by general malaise
II. **Clinical Features:** Each of the following symptoms is frequently associated with colds, flu, and upper respiratory infections (URIs) and is discussed separately:
   A. Sore throat
   B. Cough
   C. Nasal congestion
   D. Sinusitis
   E. Allergy/hay fever
   F. Diarrhea
   G. Nausea/vomiting
III. **Management**
   A. Increase rest
   B. Increase fluids
   C. Humidifier, vaporizer
   D. For general aches and pains, take Tylenol 1 or 2 every four hours as needed.
   E. Over-the-counter (OTC) medications, such as Actifed and Sudafed, contain multiple ingredients. None have shown harmful effects on the fetus but the use of multiple ingredient compounds should be discouraged. NaCl gargles; Robitussin for cough.
   F. Optional: vitamin C, 2 to 5 gm a day, divided into equal dosages every 3 to 4 hours. If toxicity symptoms occur (eg, slight burning during urination, loose bowels, gas retention and/or skin rashes), reduce dosage.

NOTES

COUGHS

I. **Clinical Features**
   A. History
      1. Onset, duration, course, any self-treatment measures?
      2. Is patient a smoker?
      3. Previous history of coughs?
      4. Any sputum? If so, what is the color? Is it bloody?
      5. Associated signs and symptoms
         a. Nasal congestion
         b. Fever, myalgia
         c. Nausea/vomiting
         d. Headache
         e. Lung involvement
         f. Sore throat
   B. Physical exam
      1. Inspect throat for infection, edema, abscess. Differentiate between infection and irritation from coughing.
      2. Palpate submental, submaxillar, tonsillar, and cervical lymph nodes. If swollen and tender, indicative of infection.
      3. Percuss and auscultate lungs for decreased breath sounds, wheezes, rales, rhonchi, areas of consolidation. If present, indicative of lung involvement.
      4. Take temperature. If elevated, indicative of infection.
   C. Labwork
      1. If throat infected, obtain culture.
      2. CBC and other labwork as necessary.

II. **Management**
   A. Lemon and honey mixed together and used as cough syrup
   B. OTC cough syrups
      1. Robitussin plain or DM
      2. Phenergan expectorant
   C. Saline or mouthwash gargle
   D. Throat lozenges (or hard candy)
   E. If severe:
      1. Robitussin AC
      2. Nucofed
      3. Practitioner's choice
   F. If cough persists more than 7 days:
      1. Reassess, consider a chest radiograph.
      2. Rule out pneumonia, tuberculosis, allergies, asthma.

3. For treatment of uncomplicated productive cough, prescribe an antibiotic.
G. Consult physician in the following situations:
1. Chronic cough or cough that does not respond to measures listed above.
2. Clinical picture that is suggestive of pneumonia.

NOTES

DIABETES MELLITUS

I. **Definition:** A chronic disorder that is characterized by hyperglycemia, associated with major abnormalities in carbohydrate, fat, and protein metabolism. Patients with diabetes have a tendency to develop renal, ocular, neurologic, and premature cardiovascular diseases.

II. **Incidence:** Approximately 3 in 100 pregnancies

III. **Etiology**
   A. Glucose metabolism in pregnancy
      1. The pregnant woman has fasting hypoglycemia because the baby uses glucose from the mother's bloodstream at a constant rate. The pregnant woman may have hypoglycemia symptoms because the normal fasting blood sugar (FBS) in pregnancy is 65.
      2. The pregnant woman has postprandial (PP) hyperglycemia because of elevation of certain hormones that antagonize insulin and make it less effective.
         a. Human placental lactogen
         b. Cortisol
         c. Estrogen
         d. Progesterone
   B. Insulin requirements change throughout pregnancy.
      1. In the first 20 weeks, insulin requirements drop because:
         a. The baby is using glucose from the mother's bloodstream at a constant rate, yet the hormones that antagonize insulin are not yet being produced in significant amounts.
         b. Nausea and vomiting are common, so the woman's food intake may be less than normal.
      2. There is an ever-increasing need for insulin in the last 20 weeks. If the woman's pancreas cannot produce this extra insulin, the glucose from the food she eats cannot be used by her cells, resulting in hyperglycemia and ketosis.
   C. Effect on the fetus
      1. Because of hyperglycemia in the diabetic mother, the baby's pancreas is stimulated to hyperinsulinism, which enhances glycogen synthesis, lipogenesis, and protein synthesis, leading to macrosomia.
      2. The woman may be relatively asymptomatic because it is common for pregnant women to complain of hunger, thirst, and polyuria. Yet without treatment, the baby is in jeopardy. Besides macrosomia, there is an increased incidence of perinatal complications, such as:
         a. Stillbirths
         b. Birth trauma
         c. Neonatal hypoglycemia

IV. **Clinical Features**
   A. Classification

1. Class A: Gestational
   a. Diabetes mellitus induced by pregnancy, diagnosed on the basis of an abnormal glucose tolerance test (GTT)
   b. Blood sugar returns to normal after the pregnancy ends.
   c. 20% of average weight and 60% of overweight patients with gestational diabetes will develop diabetes mellitus later in life.
2. Class B: Overt, adult onset
   a. Onset after age 20
   b. Duration less than 10 years
   c. No evidence of vascular disease
3. Class C: Overt, teen onset
   a. Duration 10 to 19 years
   b. No evidence of vascular disease
4. Class D: Overt, childhood onset
   a. Onset under age 10
   b. Duration more than 20 years
   c. Calcification of the vessels of the leg
   d. Benign retinopathy
   e. Hypertension

B. History
   1. Family history of diabetes
   2. Two or more spontaneous abortions
   3. Stillbirth or unexplained neonatal death
   4. Giving birth to a baby with macrosomia (>9.6 lbs, 4500 gm)
   5. Giving birth to a baby with congenital anomalies
   6. Polyhydramnios in a previous pregnancy
   7. Hypertensive disorders in a previous pregnancy
   8. Predisposition to infections, especially UTIs and monilia vaginitis

C. Contributing factors in present pregnancy:
   1. Obesity—any of the following:
      a. Being more than 30% overweight at the beginning of the pregnancy
      b. Reaching 200 pounds at any time in the pregnancy
      c. Large weight gain in pregnancy (see Weight Gain in Pregnancy on page 31)
   2. Glycosuria
   3. Polyhydramnios
   4. Hypertension
   5. Multiple gestation
   6. Frequent infections, especially UTIs and monilia vaginitis

V. **Diagnosis**

A. Fifty percent of class A diabetics can be diagnosed by history.

1. Presence of one or more predisposing factors
2. Signs and symptoms of diabetes
    a. Polyuria (excessive urinary output)
    b. Polydipsia (excessive thirst)
    c. Polyphagia (excessive hunger)
    d. Unexplained weight loss, especially in the presence of a large food intake. Or may see unexplained weight gain in the presence of a normal food intake.
    e. Weakness
B. The other 50% can be picked up by lab tests.
    1. Glycosuria on two consecutive occasions not related to carbohydrate intake warrants further investigation.
        a. One in 10 such women have class A diabetes.
        b. The other 9 in 10 have glycosuria of pregnancy due to decreased kidney threshold for glucose.
    2. FBS and 2-hour PP BS, 1 hour post 50 gm glucola load BS, and 3-hour GTT are other lab tests to assess carbohydrate metabolism. Abnormal levels are diagnostic of diabetes.
        a. When done at 20 weeks, 60% to 80% of women with class A diabetes will be detected.
        b. When done at 26 weeks, an even greater percentage will be detected.
        c. If only one test can be done, 24 to 26 weeks' gestation is the optimum compromise time.
C. Overt diabetes is diagnosed on the basis of two or more FBSs of 105 or greater, two or more elevated values on a GTT, or 1-hour glucola above 200.

VI. **Management**
   A. Lab tests
      1. Test the urine at each routine prenatal visit.
         a. If there is glycosuria, question the patient about her recent intake of refined carbohydrates.
         b. If only a trace glycosuria and positive diet history.
            (1) Counsel regarding avoidance of refined carbohydrates.
            (2) Recheck at next visit.
         c. If more than trace glycosuria times two, not diet-related schedule for either a FBS and 2-hour PP BS or a 1-hour post 50-gm glucola load BS (see section A-3 below).
      2. On all pregnant patients, order a glucola load BS or a 2-hour PP BS after a 50- or 100-gm high carbohydrate diet for patients unable to do 50-gm loading dose.
         a. Preferably between 24 and 28 weeks
         b. Immediately in the following situations:
            (1) History of stillborn or unexplained neonatal death
            (2) History of gestational diabetes

(3) Sibling or parent with insulin-dependent diabetes
(4) Two consecutive episodes of glycosuria unrelated to carbohydrate intake
(5) Strong suspicion of diabetes, based on two or more predisposing factors, presence of symptoms, or both

3. Order a 3-hour GTT and a hemoglobin AIC if abnormal results are obtained from either a FBS, 2-hour PP BS or a 1-hour post 50-gm glucola load BS as ordered in #2 above. Results are considered abnormal if the following values are met or exceeded.
   a. FBS: 105 mg glucose/100 ml plasma
   b. 2-hour PP: 120
   c. 1-hour post 50 gm glucola: 140
   d. GTT
      (1) FBS: 105
      (2) 1-hour: 195
      (3) 2-hour: 165
      (4) 3-hour: 145

B. Diagnosis is made on the basis of an abnormal GTT.
   1. If the GTT is grossly abnormal, the patient should be referred for physician management.
   2. If the GTT is mildly abnormal (2 abnormal values, none above 200) consult with physician. Collaborative management is possible. Usual course:
      a. Put the patient on a 2200 to 2400 caloric diabetic diet. Offer referral to a dietitian. Tips for diet:
         (1) Eat 150 to 200 gm carbohydrates (CHO) per day.
            (a) Eat only complex CHO: starches, bread, pasta, beans, potatoes.
            (b) Avoid all refined CHO: eat very little fruit.
            (c) Divide food evenly throughout the day; eat regular meals and snacks. Eat two sevenths of CHO in morning, two sevenths at lunch, two sevenths at dinner, and one seventh at bedtime.
         (2) Eat 100 to 150 gm protein per day.
         (3) Eat 45 to 90 gm fat per day or about 35% of total calories.

C. Continuing management
   1. When possible, refer for home glucose/urine monitoring.
   2. Schedule the patient for a FBS and 2-hour PP BS after 2 weeks of being on the diet. The meal for the 2-hour PP BS should be the usual diabetic meal, not a high carbohydrate meal.
      a. If the blood sugars are normal, the patient can continue to be comanaged. About two thirds of women will be in this category.
      b. If the blood sugars are abnormal, consult. Physician referral is probably indicated.

c. Start strict fetal activity count at 30 weeks.

d. Nonstress test (NST) weekly after 32 to 34 weeks, biweekly after 36 weeks

e. Plan to deliver baby at 39–40 weeks before it is too large.

VII. **Complications** (seldom seen in class A diabetes)
   A. Maternal
   1. Polyhydramnios is common for unknown reasons; it can lead to premature rupture of membranes, respiratory distress.
   2. The likelihood of pre-eclampsia is increased times four.
   3. Infection occurs more often and is likely to be more severe.
   4. Caesarean section is much more common due to fetal macrosomia, fetal distress, and worsening of condition in the last weeks of pregnancy.
   5. Postpartum hemorrhage is more common.
   6. Vascular complications (eg, proliferating retinopathy and nephropathy), especially in diabetics of long duration
   B. Fetal
   1. Intrauterine fetal death
      a. Incidence: 3% to 12%
   2. Neonatal morbidity
      a. Incidence: 4% to 7%
      b. Causes
         (1) Hyperbilirubinemia—possibly due to prematurity
         (2) Macrosomia—may cause birth injury if delivery is vaginal.
         (3) Hypoglycemia—due to sudden withdrawal of maternal hyperglycemia
         (4) Hypocalcemia—due to asphyxia, prematurity, or a variety of other possibilities
         (5) Idiopathic respiratory distress. Contributing factors:
            (a) High incidence of caesareans
            (b) Desirability of delivery before term to lessen mortality
            (c) Babies of diabetic mothers make a different, less efficient type of surfactant. The lecithin/spingomyelin (LS) ratio, which normally indicates lung maturity at 2:1, may be unreliable.
   3. Fetal morbidity: 5% to 10% of those above class A have congenital malformations versus 3% normally; most common are ventral septal defects and neural disorders.

DIARRHEA

I. **Etiology**
   A. Viral, bacterial, or protozoan
      1. Sometimes related to flu syndrome (see Colds, Flu, Upper Respiratory Infection on page 99).
      2. Gastroenteritis
   B. Related to diet
   C. Sometimes due to lactose intolerance, especially in dark-skinned races
   D. Associated with antibiotic therapy
   E. Contaminated water, new puppy *(Giardia)*

II. **Management**
   A. Acute onset—history:
      1. Elicit onset, severity, whether other family members have had it, what measures have been taken to relieve it, whether other symptoms are present.
      2. Diet history
         a. Any recent change in eating habits?
         b. Seasonal, for example, access to fresh fruits or vegetables
         c. Eating bran, other whole grains, beans, or other legumes?
         d. Could contaminated dairy products, eggs, meat, and so on have been consumed?
         e. Determine if recent increase in dairy products due to pregnancy, or history of lactose intolerance in family. If so, may try acidophilus-cultured milk or adding lactase to dairy products.
      3. Taking large doses of vitamin C? If so, reduce dosage—may be causing diarrhea.
   B. Acute onset—management
      1. Avoid dairy products for 24 hours.
      2. Maintain a clear liquid diet for 24 hours.
      3. Take Kaopectate, Imodium AD, or Pepto-Bismol as needed. May need Lomotil if severe.
      4. If abdominal cramping: take one Phazyme before each meal and one at bedtime.
      5. Check for ketonuria. Advise patient to check her urine 2 hours after eating. If more than a trace of ketonuria for over 48 hours, she should call.
      6. If unrelieved in 48 hours, get stool specimen for ova and parasites
      7. If *Giardia* is present, treat with Flagyl, 250 mg orally three times a day for 5 to 7 days or 375 mg orally twice a day for 7 days
      8. Consult with physician if:
         a. Diarrhea persists despite treatment.
         b. Significant dehydration is present.

c. Ketonuria is unrelieved in 24 hours.
C. Chronic
   1. Ascertain whether prenatal vitamins contain a stool softener. If so, try a vitamin without a stool softener.
   2. Consult with physician, may be colitis, etc.

NOTES

DYSFUNCTIONAL UTERINE BLEEDING

I. **Definition:** Abnormal uterine bleeding with no demonstrable or organic cause. It is a diagnosis of exclusion.
II. **Incidence**
   A. Fifty percent are 40 to 50 years old.
   B. Twenty percent are adolescents.
III. **Etiology**
   A. Anovulation is most common cause.
   B. Coagulation defects
   C. Perimenopausal patients
      1. Shortening of proliferative phase
      2. Corpus luteum dysfunction
IV. **Laboratory**
   A. Pap smear, endometrial biopsy, QBHCG, CBC, coagulation studies, TSH, FSH, and DHEAS if masculinization is present
   B. Ultrasound
V. **Differential Diagnosis**
   A. Pathology of pregnancy
      1. Ectopic
         a. Positive HCG
         b. Unilateral pain
         c. Bleeding
      2. Abortion
         a. Threatened
         b. Incomplete
         c. Missed
      3. Trophoblastic disease—very high QBHCG
      4. Postpartum
         a. Subinvolution
         b. Retained products of conception
         c. Infection
   B. Malignancy
      1. Cervical cancer
      2. Uterine cancer
      3. Fallopian tube cancer
   C. Chronic endometritis
      1. Episodic intermenstrual spotting
      2. TB endometritis
   D. Uterine defects
      1. Fibroids

2. Endometrial polyps
 E. Pathology of cervix, vagina, and ovaries
    1. Cervical polyps
    2. Severe vaginal infections
    3. Corpus luteum dysfunction
    4. Ovarian tumors, especially hormone secreting
 F. Systemic diseases
    1. Coagulation defects
       a. von Willebrand's disease
       b. Leukemias
       c. Severe sepsis
    2. Hypothyroidism—elevated TSH
    3. Adrenal insufficiency
       a. Usually causes oligomenorrhea or amenorrhea
       b. Rarely causes irregular vaginal bleeding
    4. Cirrhosis
       a. Reduced capacity of liver to metabolize estrogens
       b. Can also have hypoprothrombinemia
    5. Iatrogenic causes
       a. Birth control pills
       b. Depo-Provera
       c. Hormone replacement therapy (HRT)
       d. Danazol
       e. GnRH Agonist
          (1) Synarel
          (2) Lupron
       f. Tranquilizers
       g. IUDs

VI. **Management**
 A. Evaluation
    1. History and physical
    2. Question last menstrual period (LMP), previous menstrual period (PMP), dysmenorrhea, menorrhagia.
    3. Pregnancy
    4. Contraception
    5. Trauma
 B. Possible therapies
    1. Birth control pills (BCPs)
    2. Provera
    3. Premarin/Provera
    4. Clomid if pregnancy desired
 C. Refer as appropriate.

1. Hysteroscopy
2. Dilation and curettage (D&C)
3. Uterine ablation
4. Hysterectomy with or without bilateral salpingostomatomies

NOTES

DYSMENORRHEA

I. **Definition**
   A. Primary dysmenorrhea: Painful menstruation unrelated to an obvious physical cause.
   B. Secondary dysmenorrhea: Demonstrable pelvic disease is present.

II. **Incidence**
   A. Occurs to some degree in 40% to 80% of all women.
   B. Is so severe that it is incapacitating in 5% to 10%.

III. **Etiology**
   A. Primary dysmenorrhea
      1. Believed to be caused by high endometrial levels of prostaglandins. Under the influence of progesterone during the luteal phase of the menstrual cycle, the endometrial content of prostaglandins is increased, reaching a maximum at the onset of menstruation.
      2. Prostaglandins cause strong myometrial contractions that constrict the blood vessels, resulting in ischemia, endometrial disintegration, bleeding, and pain.
   B. Secondary dysmenorrhea may be caused by any of the following:
      1. Endometriosis
      2. Uterine polyps or fibroids
      3. PID
      4. Dysfunctional uterine bleeding
      5. Uterine prolapse
      6. Maladaptation to an IUD
      7. Retained products of conception following spontaneous abortion (SAB), therapeutic abortion (TAB), or childbirth
      8. Uterine, ovarian cancer

IV. **Clinical Features**
   A. Primary dysmenorrhea
      1. Description of course
         a. Presents as low, midline cramping, spasmodic in nature, may radiate to back or inner thighs.
         b. Discomfort commonly begins 1 or 2 days before the onset of flow, but pain is characteristically most severe during the first 24 hours of flow and subsides by the second day.
         c. Frequently accompanied by side effects such as:
            (1) Vomiting
            (2) Diarrhea
            (3) Headache
            (4) Syncope
            (5) Leg pains
      2. Characteristics and associated factors:
         a. Characteristically begins 1 to 3 years after menarche

- **b.** Increases in severity over several years to ages 23 to 27, then begins to decline.
- **c.** More common in nulliparous women; frequently decreases significantly after the birth of a child
- **d.** More common in obese women
- **e.** Associated with a prolonged menstrual flow
- **f.** Less common in athletes
- **g.** Less common in women who have irregular cycles

B. Secondary dysmenorrhea
1. Suspect if:
   - **a.** Dysmenorrhea begins after the age of 20.
   - **b.** The pain is unilateral.
2. Associated factors according to cause:
   - **a.** PID
     - (1) Acute onset
     - (2) Frequently involves dyspareunia.
     - (3) Tenderness to palpation and on movement
     - (4) There may be a palpable adnexal mass.
   - **b.** Endometriosis
     - (1) Cyclic dyspareunia
     - (2) Pain does not precede the flow and does not end within a few hours as in primary. Instead, it increases in intensity throughout the period.
     - (3) Pain is steady rather than crampy and may be specific to the lesion site.
     - (4) Occasionally, nodules may be palpated on exam.
   - **c.** Uterine fibroids and polyps
     - (1) Onset of dysmenorrhea is later in the reproductive years than primary.
     - (2) Frequently accompanied by changes in the menstrual flow.
     - (3) Characterized by a cramping pain
     - (4) Fibroids may be palpated.
     - (5) Polyps may or may not be protruding from the cervix.
   - **d.** Uterine prolapse
     - (1) Onset is later in the reproductive years than primary dysmenorrhea.
     - (2) More common in multipara patients
     - (3) Tends to manifest as backache beginning premenstrually and persisting through the period
     - (4) Often accompanied by dyspareunia and pelvic pain, which are more severe premenstrually and may be relieved by recumbent or knee-chest position.
     - (5) Found concurrently with cystocele and urinary stress incontinence

C. Differentiate according to history and physical exam.
   1. History
      a. Menstrual history
         (1) Onset of menarche
         (2) Onset of dysmenorrhea in relation to menarche
         (3) Frequency and regularity of cycles
         (4) Duration and amount of flow
         (5) Relationship of dysmenorrhea to cycle and flow
      b. Description of pain
         (1) Onset in relation to menstrual period
         (2) Cramping, spasmodic, steady
         (3) Generalized or in a specific location
         (4) Unilateral or all over lower abdomen
         (5) Location: lower abdomen, back, thighs
         (6) Worse on palpation or movement
      c. Associated symptoms
         (1) Extragenital symptoms (see section IV. A-1-c)
         (2) Dyspareunia—relationship to menstrual cycle constant or cyclical
      d. Obstetric history—parity
      e. Is there an IUD in place?
      f. Any history of conditions that may result in secondary dysmenorrhea?
   2. Physical exam
      a. Note age, weight.
      b. Speculum exam
         (1) Observe for polyps at the os.
         (2) Note unusual color or odor of discharge, do a wet prep.
         (3) Cervical culture plus STD cultures and blood work as necessary by history
      c. Bimanual exam
         (1) Note cervical motion tenderness.
         (2) Note size, shape, and consistency of uterus; feel for fibroids.
         (3) Note adnexal mass or nodules.
         (4) Note uterine or adnexal tenderness, especially unilateral.
         (5) Note cystocele, uterine prolapse.

V. **Management**
   A. For primary dysmenorrhea
      1. Exercise
         a. Moderate exercise, such as a walk or swim

b. Pelvic rocking exercises
   c. Lying with knees to chest on back or side
2. Heat
   a. Heating pad or hot water bottle to lower back or lower abdomen
   b. Hot bath, shower, or sauna
3. Orgasm relieves pelvic congestion. Warning: intercourse without orgasm may increase pelvic congestion.
4. Avoid caffeine, which can increase release of prostaglandins.
5. Massage of back, leg, or calf
6. Rest
7. Drugs
   a. Oral contraceptives inhibit ovulation and thus relieve the symptoms.
   b. The Progestasert IUD may prevent cramping.
   c. Drug of choice: Ibuprofen 200 to 800 mg orally every 4 to 12 hours depending on dosage, Aleve 200 orally every 6 hours, etc.

B. For secondary dysmenorrhea
   1. PID
      a. PID may include endometritis, salpingitis, tubo-ovarian abscess, or pelvic peritonitis.
      b. Causative organisms often include *N. gonorrhoeae* and *C. trachomatis,* as well as gram-negatives, anaerobes, group B streptococcus, and genital mycoplasmas. Take appropriate cultures.
      c. Treatment with broad-spectrum antibiotics should begin as soon as the diagnosis is made to prevent permanent damage (ie, adhesions, sterility, etc.).
         (1) For serious cases, consider consultation to hospitalize for a course of IV antibiotics.
         (2) Cefoxitin 2 g IM plus probenecid 1 g orally (ceftiaxone 250 mg IM or equivalent cephalosporin), plus doxycycline 100 mg orally, twice daily for 10 to 14 days.
         (3) If unable to tolerate doxycycline, give erythromycin 500 gm, orally four times a day for 10 to 14 days.
      d. IUD, although the effect of removal of an IUD on response to treatment is unknown, removal is recommended.
   2. Endometriosis
      a. Confirmatory diagnosis needs to be made by laparoscope.
      b. May treat with BCPs, Lupron, etc., as directed by the physician
   3. Uterine fibroids and polyps
      a. Cervical polyps need to be removed.
      b. Symptomatic uterine fibroids need to be referred to a physician.

4. Uterine prolapse
   a. Definitive treatment; refer for hysterectomy
   b. Concurrent cystocele/urinary stress incontinence
      (1) Kegel's exercises
      (2) Pessary and introl devices to reposition and raise the bladder, may offer some relief.

NOTES

ECTOPIC PREGNANCY

I. **Definition:** Implantation of the blastocyst anywhere besides the endometrium. The site is usually in the most distal part of the fallopian tube.

II. **Incidence:** Occurs in 1 in 200 pregnancies in white women, 1 in 120 pregnancies in nonwhite women. Recurs in 7% to 20% of cases.

III. **Etiology**
   A. Conditions that prevent or retard passage of the fertilized ovum to the uterus:
      1. Endosalpingitis (PID)
      2. Developmental anomalies
      3. Adhesions in the tube from previous surgeries, infections, IUD
      4. Tumors that distort the shape of the tube.
      5. Menstrual reflux
      6. Hormonal factors that slow peristalsis of the tube.
   B. Increase in receptivity of the tubal mucosa of the fertilized ovum (eg, endometriosis)

IV. **Clinical Course:** If not diagnosed and removed, will eventually rupture. Signs and symptoms are:
   A. Before rupture
      1. Amenorrhea, then continuous intermittent spotting. May be subtle, so that the spotting appears to be a normal menstrual period.
      2. Pelvic, abdominal pain, sometimes neck/shoulder pain
      3. Soft pliable mass palpated in adnexa. Mass may be firm if distended with blood.
      4. Uterus does enlarge due to the placental hormones, may be normal size for gestation. May be displaced to one side.
      5. Nausea, vomiting less common than usual. Diarrhea more common than usual.
      6. Positive pregnancy test but may be negative up to 50% of the time due to suboptimal placental function.
      7. Acute abdominal pain—may be anywhere in the abdomen.
   B. After rupture:
      1. Sudden, severe, sharp, lower abdominal pain
      2. Hypotension and signs of shock depending on amount of internal bleeding; can lose large amounts quickly.
      3. Abdominal pain and cervical motion tenderness
      4. Blood in the cul-de-sac
      5. Pain in the neck and shoulder, especially on inspiration, due to irritation of diaphragm from blood in the peritoneal cavity

V. **Differential Diagnosis**
   A. Spontaneous abortion
      1. More bleeding

       2. Less pain
       3. No adnexal mass palpated
       4. Lower incidence of shock
       5. Products of conception may be expelled and found on speculum exam or in the toilet.
    B. PID
       1. History of previous infection
       2. Amenorrhea rare
       3. Pain is bilateral, not unilateral
       4. Fever usually greater than 101°F
    C. Ovarian cyst
       1. Normal menses
       2. Pain uncommon
       3. Mass smooth and mobile
       4. Uterus feels nonpregnant.
    D. Appendicitis
       1. Nausea, vomiting, fever almost always present
       2. No signs and symptoms of pregnancy
       3. Pelvic exam normal
       4. Pain in epigastrium, not neck and shoulder
       5. Presence of McBurney's sign

VI. **Management**
    A. See Guidelines for Bleeding Under 20 Weeks' Gestation on page 85.
    B. Ultrasound
    C. See that all unsensitized Rh(D)–negative patients receive Rh(D) immune globulin, 1 vial, IM within 72 hours of rupture or removal to prevent possible sensitization from an Rh(D) positive fetus.
    D. Treatment is always surgical. Refer to physician.
    E. Inform patient that there is a 7% to 20% risk for repeat ectopic pregnancy.

EDEMA IN PREGNANCY

I. **Etiology**
   A. High estrogen levels make the blood vessels more fragile and "leaky."
   B. Impaired venous circulation and increased venous pressure in the lower extremities due to:
      1. Pressure of the enlarging uterus on the pelvic veins when sitting or standing.
      2. Pressure of the enlarging uterus on the vena cava when supine.
   C. Increased venous pressure may also be due to the expanding blood volume of pregnancy.

II. **Clinical Features**
   A. Physiologic edema is dependent.
      1. Usually seen in the feet and ankles after being upright, and decreases with leg elevation or bedrest.
      2. May be seen in the sacrum if on bedrest
      3. Not usually seen in the face or hands
   B. Very common in pregnancy and may be a sign of well-being because it indicates an expanding blood volume

III. **Differential Diagnosis**
   A. Pre-eclampsia
      1. Usually more severe than physiologic edema
      2. Sudden onset
      3. Generalized body edema, particularly in face and hands
      4. Present even after bedrest, limb elevation, or both
      5. Look for other signs and symptoms:
         a. High blood pressure
         b. Proteinuria
         c. Brisk deep tendon reflexes (DTRs)
         d. Elevated hematocrit, decreased platelets
   B. High sodium intake. Salt should not be restricted during pregnancy, but consuming an excessive amount may result in edema.
      1. May see generalized, nondependent edema
      2. History of high sodium intake from foods such as ham, potato chips, pretzels; habit of oversalting food

IV. **Management**
   A. When a patient presents with edema, make a differential diagnosis.
      1. Assess characteristics of edema.
         a. Onset
         b. Severity
         c. Relieved by bedrest, limb elevation, or both
      2. Diet history: recent high sodium intake
      3. History of prolonged standing or sitting

4. Habit of wearing tight waistbands or stockings, which further constrict the circulation
5. Look for signs and symptoms of pre-eclampsia.
- **B.** If diagnosis is physiologic edema:
  1. Avoid constrictive clothing.
  2. Lie down and elevate legs periodically throughout the day to aid venous return.
  3. Elastic stockings may aid venous return. Put them on before arising in the morning.
  4. Take rest periods lying on the left side to keep the uterus off the vena cava and aid venous return.
  5. Avoid excessive sodium in the diet.
  6. Call office if edema suddenly becomes more severe or generalized, in spite of the above measures.

NOTES

ENDOMETRIAL BIOPSY

I. **Definition:** Obtaining a sample of the endometrial lining to screen for endometrial cancer or hyperplasia.

II. **Indications**
   A. Irregular uterine bleeding of unknown etiology in a woman of 35 years or older
   B. Presence of any vaginal bleeding in a postmenopausal woman.
   C. Screening of woman before initiating HRT. Routine screening is controversial; some recommend rescreening patients with HRT every 1 to 2 years.
   D. Staging of the endometrium of the infertile patient, or patient with recurrent fetal wastage, to diagnose luteal phase defect.

III. **Contraindications**
   A. Pregnancy
   B. PID

IV. **Technique**
   A. Giving 600 to 800 mg orally of ibuprofen or some other antiprostaglandin 20 to 30 minutes before procedure may be of benefit. If desired, an antibiotic may be given prophylactically before and 6 to 8 hours after the procedure.
   B. Select one of several instruments designed for endometrial sampling. The pipelle endometrial suction curette is described here. It is a disposable, flexible curette, 23.5 cm long with color markings at 4, 7, 8, and 10 cm from the end.
   C. Perform a bimanual exam to determine size, shape, and position of the uterus.
   D. Visualize the cervix, clean with an antiseptic. If desired or necessary, the cervix may be straightened by grasping with a tenaculum. A sound may be introduced to determine the length of the uterus. Gently introduce the pipelle up into the uterine fundus. Pull the piston of the pipelle back, creating a negative pressure while rotating 360 degrees as the pipelle is moved from the fundus toward the os. Tissue being collected should be seen within the sheath.

V. **Complications:** Rare and reported to be below 1 per 1000.
   A. Infection may be prevented by pre- and post-medication with a broad spectrum antibiotic.
   B. Bleeding
   C. Potential perforation of the uterus (there are no reported cases using the pipelle)

VI. **Management**
   A. Benign: Proliferative or secretory
      1. BCPs
      2. Cycle with Provera or other progestational agent
   B. Cystic or adenomatous hyperplasia

1. Desires pregnancy: Induce ovulation. If not pregnant within 6 months, repeat endometrial biopsy.
2. Pregnancy not desired/postmenopausal
    a. Remove unopposed estrogen source by cycling with BCPs or Provera 10 mg orally starting days 14 to 16 of period for 10 to 12 days each menstrual cycle. Megace or other progestational agent may be used.
    b. Repeat endometrial biopsy in 6 months.
        (1) If normal, continue to follow.
        (2) If hyperplasia, refer for D&C, possible hysterectomy.
C. Atypical adenomatous hyperplasia: refer to physician.

NOTES

ENDOMETRITIS

I. **Definition:** Infection of the endometrium, decidua, and myometrium of the uterus after delivery.
II. **Etiology**
   A. Bacteria invade the area after delivery and spread rapidly.
   B. Sources of bacteria may be any one or a combination of:
      1. Endogenous vaginal bacteria, usually pathogenic only when tissue is damaged or devitalized
         a. Beta hemolytic streptococcus
         b. *Streptococcus viridans*
         c. *Neisseria gonococcus*
         d. *Gardnerella*
      2. Contamination by normal bowel bacteria
         a. *Clostridium welchii*
         b. *Escherichia coli*
         c. *Proteus mirabilis*
         d. *Aerobacter aerogenes*
         e. *Enterococcus*
         f. *Pseudomonas aeruginosa*
         g. *Klebsiella pneumonia*
      3. Contamination from environment. Staphylococcus is a common organism.
III. **Clinical Features**
   A. Predisposing causes
      1. Extensive tissue edema
      2. Prolonged labor
      3. Prolonged rupture of membranes
      4. Numerous vaginal exams in labor
      5. Breaks in aseptic technique
      6. Careless handwashing
      7. Any intrauterine manipulation: placement of intrauterine catheter, internal rotation, or manual removal of the placenta.
      8. Retained placental fragments or membranes
      9. Operative delivery
      10. Improper perineal care, leading to contamination by gastrointestinal bacteria
      11. Malnutrition, debilitation, anemia, excessive blood loss, preexisting infection
   B. Signs and symptoms
      1. Fever and chills
         a. Fever between 100.4°F and 104°F, depending on severity of infection

b. Temperature is often low grade for several days then spikes.
c. Chills indicate severe infection.
2. Tachycardia between 100 and 140, depending on severity of infection
3. Uterine signs and symptoms
   a. Tenderness extending laterally
   b. Prolonged or recurrent afterbirth pains
   c. Subinvolution
   d. Slight abdominal distention
   e. Abnormalities of lochia
      (1) May be scant and odorless if anaerobic infection
      (2) May be moderately heavy, foul, bloody, seropurulent if aerobic infection
4. Onset usually 3 to 5 days after delivery unless caused by beta hemolytic streptococcus. Then onset is earlier and more precipitous.
5. Elevated WBC more than usual for postpartum; greater than 25,000

IV. **Differential Diagnosis** (See Puerperal Infection Guidelines on page 212.)

V. **Management**
   A. If history/signs/symptoms consistent with endometritis:
      1. Perform sterile speculum exam.
         a. Observe character and odor of lochia.
         b. Obtain cultures as necessary of cervix and to rule out STDs.
      2. Perform sterile bimanual exam.
         a. Assess uterus for unusual tenderness
         b. Assess uterus for bogginess.
      3. Obtain CBC if febrile.
      4. Antibiotic treatment pending culture results:
         a. Ampicillin 500 mg orally four times a day for 10 days if not allergic
         b. If allergic to penicillin and not breastfeeding, doxycycline 100 mg orally every 12 hours for 7 days
         c. If allergic to penicillin and breastfeeding, Keflex 500 mg orally four times a day for 7 days.
      5. If uterus boggy and/or bleeding excessive, prescribe Methergine 0.2 mg orally every 4 hours for six doses. **Do not** give Methergine if patient is hypertensive.
      6. Instruct patient to take temperature four times a day for the next week. It should be below 100°F within 48 hours of starting antibiotics.
      7. Instruct patient to drink 3 liters of fluid daily and increase rest.
      8. Obtain results of cultures, both preliminary and final. Patient needs to be on antibiotic to which organism is sensitive. Check safety of antibiotic during breastfeeding.
      9. Patient should be instructed to call if symptoms do not resolve within 24 hours, or if they worsen. If no significant improvement

within 2 to 3 days, patient may need to be admitted to hospital for treatment. Otherwise, follow up by telephone or office visit within 3 days.
- **C.** Consult with physician in the following situations:
    1. Symptoms do not resolve or worsen within 24 hours.
    2. Temperature does not go below 100°F after 48 hours on antibiotics.
- **D.** Prevention and early detection of endometritis
    1. Encourage good nutrition during pregnancy.
    2. Prevent or treat anemia.
    3. Try to avoid overexhaustion in labor.
    4. If membranes have ruptured:
        a. Confirm with a sterile speculum exam unless in active labor.
        b. Do not perform vaginal exams if there is no labor.
        c. Minimize vaginal exams as much as possible if the patient is in active labor.
    5. Avoid unnecessary vaginal exams whether membranes are ruptured or not.
    6. Take patient's temperature at least every 4 hours in active labor, every 2 hours if membranes are ruptured.
    7. Observe careful aseptic technique.
        a. Keep field as sterile as possible.
        b. Place a sterile drape under patient's hips before delivery.
        c. Avoid rectal contamination of the vaginal area.
        d. Change gloves between delivery of the baby and internal inspection and suturing.
    8. Assess placenta for intactness.
        a. Watch for signs of infection if possible retained fragments or membranes.
        b. Do uterine exploration if probable retained fragments or membranes.
    9. Avoid extensive manipulation of tissue while suturing.
    10. Instruct patient in good perineal care.
        a. Wipe from front to back.
        b. Remove peri pad from front to back.
        c. Change peri pad at least every 4 hours.
        d. Wash vulva daily and as necessary.
    11. Instruct patient in postpartum care.
        a. Take temperature four times a day for first week and call if it rises significantly or reaches 101°F.
        b. Instruct patient to call if lochia begins to smell foul, uterine tenderness develops, or cramping increases.

ESTABLISHING THE ESTIMATED DATE OF CONFINEMENT (EDC)

I. **Definition:** The estimated date of confinement (EDC) is usually 280 days, or 40 weeks after the last normal menstrual period (LNMP). It also may be calculated as 266 days, or 38 weeks from the last ovulation in a normal 28-day cycle. The EDC can be determined mathematically by using Nägele's rule: subtract three from the month of the LNMP and add 7 days.
II. **Clinical Features**
    A. History
        1. Menstrual history
            a. Length of cycles
            b. Regularity of cycles
            c. Recent menstrual history affected by:
                (1) Recent previous pregnancy, cycles not yet re-established
                (2) Breastfeeding
                (3) BCPs
                (4) Disease, trauma, other
        2. First day of last menstrual period
            a. Was it a normal period? If not, was the previous period normal?
            b. Is the exact date known, or is only a general time frame known?
        3. Contraceptive history
            a. Contraceptive method patient was using
            b. Was this method being used correctly and consistently?
        4. Sexual history
            a. Has there been regular sexual intercourse in the recent past?
            b. Have there only been isolated incidences of intercourse that could pinpoint a possible conception date?
            c. Does the patient have any idea when conception might have occurred?
        5. Fertility history
            a. Was this pregnancy planned?
            b. If so, how long did she try to conceive?
            c. What is her past pregnancy history?
        6. Symptoms of pregnancy
            a. Nausea/vomiting
            b. Breast changes, tenderness
            c. Urinary frequency
            d. Fatigue
            e. Unexplained weight gain
            f. Fetal movement

- **B.** Physical signs
    1. Bimanual palpation of uterine size in first trimester
    2. First documented FHTs
        a. Ten to twelve weeks with fetal doptone
        b. Eighteen to twenty weeks with fetascope
    3. Uterine measurements and growth trend
III. **Lab and Adjunctive Studies**
- **A.** Was a pregnancy test done? If so:
    1. When was it first positive?
    2. If ever negative, when was it last negative?
    3. Was it a urine test or a blood test?
- **B.** Sonogram: Order if dates are unclear by the above evaluation.
    1. Indications for change of menstrual EDC to ultrasound EDC:
        a. Unsure of, or had abnormal LMP
        b. Size agrees with ultrasound
        c. Ultrasound is different from LMP EDC by 7 days first trimester and 10 days until 28 weeks.

NOTES

FETAL HEART TONES

I. **Definition:** Heart tones of the fetus normally heard through the mother's abdomen. The normal rate is between 120 and 160 beats per minute.

II. **Clinical Features**
   A. FHTs can first be heard via doptone at 10 to 12 weeks.
      1. If the FHT cannot be heard with the doptone at 12 weeks by size and dates, the patient should return at 14 weeks. If at that time the FHTs are not heard, an ultrasound scan should be done to confirm fetal viability. If any abnormal results are obtained, consult with physician.
      2. FHT should be taken and recorded at every prenatal visit.
   B. FHT can first be heard via fetascope at about 18 to 20 weeks, verifying the EDC.

III. **Management: Monitoring FHT in labor**
   A. All patients should have a 10- to 15-minute fetal monitor strip on admission.
   B. Fetal monitoring should be used in the following situations:
      1. Patient request
      2. Postdates
      3. Polyhydramnios
      4. Intrauterine fetal growth retardation
      5. Hypertension
      6. Significant anemia (Hct <27%, Hbg <9.0)
      7. Unusual vaginal bleeding
      8. Abnormal fetal-placental tests (eg, low estriols, positive OCT, etc.)
      9. Premature labor
      10. Twins
      11. Abnormal FHT per auscultation or doptone
      12. Prostaglandins or prepidil for cervical ripening
      13. Pitocin induction or augmentation of labor
      14. Vaginal birth after caesarean (VBAC)
   C. The internal scalp electrode (ISE) monitor is more accurate than the external monitor.
      1. Situations in which the external monitor is adequate include:
         a. When the FHT reading via the external monitor is adequate and within normal limits
         b. Until the membranes have ruptured or until it is reasonable to rupture them to apply the internal monitor
      2. Situations in which the ISE is recommended:
         a. Non-reassuring fetal heart patterns
         b. After membranes are ruptured in all situations in section III.B
      3. Situations in which the ISE is **not** recommended, unless benefits outweigh risks:

- **a.** Bleeding disorders, for example, potential for hemophilia in the fetus, factor IX deficiency in the mother, etc.
- **b.** History of group B streptococcus, genital herpes, untreated vaginitis

D. A doptone may be used to listen to FHT in all laboring women.
1. According to the guidelines of the American College of Obstetricians and Gynecologists, FHT should be assessed in labor according to the following schedule:
    - **a.** Every 15 minutes in first stage of active labor
    - **b.** Every 5 minutes in second stage of active labor
    - **c.** More often if abnormalities are heard
2. FHTs should be listened to through a contraction and for 1 minute afterward.

NOTES

FETAL MOVEMENT

I. **Definition:** The movement of the fetus starting as early as 6 weeks. Most women do not detect it until 16 to 20 weeks gestation. Another name for the first perception of fetal movement is quickening.

II. **Clinical Features**

  A. Fetal movement should be detected by the 18th week of gestation by a multipara and by the 22nd week gestation by a primigravida.

  B. Fetal movement is highly idiosyncratic; some babies are more active than others.

  C. Babies normally have activity cycles in utero, which may correspond to sleep-awake cycles. By paying attention to the time and number of movements, the mother may become aware of a pattern of alternating stillness and activity.

  D. Smoking decreases baby's movements.

  E. Fetal movement may slow normally in amount and/or strength in the last month of pregnancy due to decreased room in the uterus, but should still occur in regular patterns and at more than 10 movements per day.

III. **Management**

  A. Near the beginning of the second trimester, ask patients if they have perceived fetal movement.

  1. If so, attempt to determine the date of quickening.

  2. If not, instruct the patient to note the date movement is first felt.

  B. The date of the first perceived fetal movement can be used to help assess the EDC.

  C. If the patient is over 24 weeks and expresses concern that the baby is not moving enough:

  1. Educate her regarding the physiologic principles of fetal activity.

  2. Have the patient count movements for 1 hour or until 10 movements have been reached.

  3. If the patient is a smoker, she needs to refrain for 1 hour.

  4. The best time to count is from 7 to 10 o'clock PM when baby is usually the most active.

  5. If the baby moves four times or more in 60 minutes, well-being is assured.

  6. If the baby moves less than four times in 60 minutes, the patient should have something to eat, drink two to three glasses of cold water, and recount for another hour. If the baby still does not move four times in 60 minutes, the patient should call.

  7. The patient should have an NST. If reactive, well-being is assured. If nonreactive, consult with physician.

  D. High-risk patients should be advised to keep a fetal movement log in the following situations:

  1. Postdates

  2. Hypertension

3. History of stillbirth or intrauterine fetal growth retardation
4. Gestational diabetes
5. FHTs heard below 120 in the office
6. At any time the patient expresses concern about fetal movement

NOTES

GALACTORRHEA

I. **Definition:** Lactation in women who have not breastfed within the past 6 months.
II. **Etiology**
   A. Physiologic
      1. Nipple stimulation
      2. Pregnancy
      3. Postpartum
   B. Pathologic
      1. Chiari-Frommel syndrome
      2. Hypothalamic disorders, hypothyroid, tumors
      3. Prolactin-secreting pituitary tumors
      4. Trauma or chronic irritation from interductal papillomas and infected milk ducts, sexual activity
   C. Pharmacologic
      1. Psychotropic drugs
      2. Antihypertensives
      3. Oral contraceptives
III. **Management**
   A. Good history and breast exam
   B. Rule out pregnancy
   C. Papanicolaou smear of breast discharge
   D. Labwork
      1. TSH—if elevated, refer for hypothyroidism
      2. Prolactin level: This level needs to be taken before the breasts are stimulated with a breast exam.
         a. Nonpregnant: less than 20 mg/ml
         b. Lactating: less than 40 mg/ml
         c. Greater than 40 to 80 mg/ml
            (1) Bromocriptine (Parlodel) 2.5 to 7.5 mg every day
            (2) Consult regarding need for computed tomography (CT) or magnetic resonance imaging (MRI) of sella turcica.
            (3) Follow with Prolactin levels every 1 to 3 months.
         d. Greater than 80 mg/ml
            (1) Order CT or MRI of sella turcica.
            (2) Refer patient to physician.
   E. Mammogram: if abnormal, refer appropriately.

GENETIC SCREENING

I. **Definition:** The process of determining the risk of genetic disorders in the fetus from the parental history and recommending appropriate testing.
II. **Etiology**
   A. Single-gene defect
      1. Autosomal dominant disorder
         a. Characteristics
            (1) An abnormal gene dominates while a normal gene is recessive.
            (2) Likelihood is 50% if a parent has the condition.
            (3) Unaffected children of affected parents are not carriers.
         b. Examples
            (1) Achondroplasia (a form of dwarfism)
            (2) Huntington's disease
            (3) Neurofibromatosis
      2. Autosomal recessive disorders
         a. Characteristics
            (1) The abnormal gene is recessive, so a gene must be contributed by each parent for offspring to be affected. Offspring who inherit one normal and one abnormal gene are carriers. All affected persons are homozygous.
            (2) If both parents are carriers, there is a 25% chance of producing either an affected child or a normal child and a 50% chance of producing a carrier.
         b. Examples
            (1) Cystic fibrosis
            (2) Sickle cell anemia
            (3) Tay-Sachs disease
            (4) Phenylketonuria
            (5) Galactosemia
      3. Sex-linked disorders
         a. Abnormal gene is carried on an X chromosome. Men are always affected. Women are affected only if both X chromosomes are abnormal, and they are carriers if one X chromosome is abnormal.
         b. Examples
            (1) Duchenne's muscular dystrophy
            (2) Hemophilia
            (3) Red-green color blindness
   B. Chromosomal aberrations
      1. Aberrations in chromosome structure: Rearrangement of genes between two paired chromosomes

2. Aberrations in chromosomal number
   a. Monosome: Cells contain one less chromosome than the basic number or aneuploid, for example, Turner's syndrome (XO).
   b. Trisomy: Cells contain three chromosomes instead of a normal pair (eg, Trisomy 21 or Down syndrome).
   c. Mosaic: Only a portion of the body cells contain the variation in chromosome number.

III. Management

A. Screening should be done at the initial visit. High risk factors include:
   1. Maternal age over 35
      a. The incidence of Down syndrome is:
         (1) Under age 25: 1 in 2000
         (2) At age 30: 1 in 885
         (3) At age 35: 1 in 250
         (4) At age 40: 1 in 109
         (5) At age 45: 1 in 12
   2. Paternal age over 55 has shown a slight increase in genetic problems.
   3. Family history of hereditary abnormality
   4. Ethnic or racial groups at high risk for specific genetic diseases:
      a. African Americans may inherit sickle cell disease or trait. Screen all African American patients for sickle cell trait.
      b. African Americans, Asians, and those of Mediterranean descent may inherit G6PD anemia. Screen only if severe or persistent anemia or UTI.
      c. People of English descent are at risk for an increased incidence of spinal cord defects.
      d. People of Jewish descent are at risk for Tay-Sachs disease.
      e. Asians and those of Mediterranean descent should be screened for thalassemia.
   5. Parents who have already had one child with a birth defect
   6. Patients who have had two or more first trimester spontaneous abortions
   7. Those with known or suspected exposure to teratogens. Ask about the following:
      a. Exposure to high temperatures (over 102°F) during the first trimester, for example, fever, hot tub, sauna. If exposed to heat during neural tube formation, spinal cord defects can result.
      b. A fever in first trimester, if caused by a viral infection, could also result in a viral-type syndrome in the fetus, such as that seen in cytomegalovirus.
      c. Primary herpes. Ask about history of herpes; if positive, ascertain whether primary episode was in first trimester.
      d. Intake of drugs since becoming pregnant, OTC, prescription, or street drugs

e. Exposure to cat litter or ingestion of raw meat
   f. Smoking increases the chance of low birth weight babies.
   g. Ingestion of alcohol. If positive, ask about fetal alcohol syndrome in present children.
   h. Caffeine intake. If excessive, recommend cutting down.
   i. Syphilis: screen if previous history.
B. Chorionic villi sampling (9–11 weeks) or amniocentesis (16–18 weeks)
   1. Should be offered in:
      a. Patients age 35 or older
      b. Parent with a chromosome abnormality
      c. Patient with previous offspring with a chromosome abnormality
      d. Parent with carrier state for metabolic disorders
      e. Parent with previous child with a neural tube defect or client with elevated serum alpha-fetoprotein (AFP)
   2. Strongly encourage such clients to make an appointment with a geneticist before deciding for or against amniocentesis. Factors in decision include:
      a. Chances of defect occurring
      b. Patient's feelings about abortions. If she would not abort the fetus regardless of defect, she may decide against amniocentesis. Even if she would not abort, knowing the diagnosis may prevent months of needless anxiety or help her prepare for parenting an affected child.
      c. Patient's feeling about defects in question. Some are more severe and/or possibly more unacceptable than others.
C. Serum AFP when estimated gestational age is 15–18 weeks. The AFP will detect between 85% to 90% of neural tube defects and 20% of Down syndrome babies. The AFP test has a false-positive rate of 30% when taken and calculated with the correct estimated gestational age.
   1. Offer to all OB patients.
   2. If elevated, ultrasound to confirm dates; repeat AFP as indicated. Refer for genetic counseling if abnormal.
   3. If decreased, ultrasound to confirm dates and AFP-plus to reconfirm a possible problem. Refer for genetics counseling and possible amniocentesis as necessary.
D. AFP-plus testing
   1. Can detect three times as many cases of Down syndrome as AFP testing alone
   2. Will detect 85% to 90% of open neural tube defects and 60% to 70% of Down syndrome babies
   3. Measures AFP, unconjugated estriol, and hCG
   4. Should be done between 15 to 18 weeks of pregnancy
      a. Offer to all patients over 35 who do not wish an amniocentesis.

b. Offer to patients who have a family history of anacephaly, neural tube defects, Down syndrome.

IV. Preventive Measures
   A. A healthy lifestyle, well-balanced meals, and avoidance of substances harmful to baby should be considered when planning pregnancy.
   B. Avoid excess vitamins; vitamin A in particular is teratogenic in high doses.
   C. Consider taking 2 to 4 mg of folic acid every day before conception to prevent neural tube defects.
   D. Avoid hot tubs, saunas, tanning beds if possibility of pregnancy.

NOTES

GONORRHEA

I. **Definition:** A sexually transmitted disease caused by an anaerobic gram-negative intracellular diplococcus, *Neisseria gonorrhoeae*.

II. **Etiology**

   A. The gonococcus (GC) organism is a kidney bean-shaped diplococcus, which is a pathogen for columnar and transactional epithelium. Common sites of infection include:
   1. Oropharynx
   2. Conjunctiva of eyes
   3. Male urethra
   4. Female reproductive tract. The GC stay in the vagina until menses when the cervical canal is open, then ascend to the uterus and tubes.
   5. Rectum

   B. Prior infection confers antibodies but no immunity. Both virulence of the bacteria and individual resistance vary.

III. **Clinical Features**

   A. Course of the disease: Onset is 3 to 7 days after first menstrual period following exposure. Symptoms begin to subside 7 to 10 days later and are usually gone after 21 days without treatment (sooner with treatment).

   B. Signs and symptoms
   1. Often asymptomatic and detected only on routine cervical screening or following possible exposure. About 40% to 60% of women with gonorrhea develop some symptoms.
   2. Urethra: Urinary frequency, slight burning on urination
   3. Paraurethral (Skene's) glands: pus can be expressed from urethral meatus.
   4. Bartholin's glands: may cause abscess (redness, edema, pain); may require incision and drainage or heal with resulting cysts.
   5. Cervix: Leukorrhea—may be green or yellow-green, irritating to vulvar tissues
   6. Endometrium: Infection is transitory, heals spontaneously and is asymptomatic.
   7. Endosalpinx: Pus forms in the tubes and can spill out onto the ovaries, peritoneum, muscle of tubes, and broad ligament. Endosalpingitis is the predominant feature of GC infection. Symptoms:
      a. Fever—up to 103°F
      b. Nausea/vomiting not uncommon
      c. Pain, moderate or severe, in both lower abdominal quadrants. Onset side may be more severe.
      d. Tenderness and rigidity in both lower abdominal quadrants on exam—involuntary guarding on abdominal palpation.

e. Cervical motion tenderness, pain in lateral fornices on bimanual exam.
f. Adnexal and/or uterine tenderness on bimanual exam
g. Adnexal mass palpated on bimanual
h. Tender inguinal adenopathy

8. Perihepatitis: Pain in the lower portion of the liver on palpation due to spread to peritoneum and fibrotic bands that form between the liver and the peritoneum.
9. Local infection: Pharyngitis, proctitis, conjunctivitis
10. Disseminated infection (arthritis-dermatitis syndrome): Spread of GC to the bloodstream.
    a. Occurs in 1% to 3% of women with gonorrhea, particularly during pregnancy or the menstrual period
    b. Is a benign condition but mimics serious conditions so must be carefully differentiated. Meningitis and endocarditis are rare.
    c. Classic triad of symptoms:
       (1) Chills and fever
       (2) Maculopapular rash on wrists and joints, which progresses to vesicles and hemorrhagic pustules.
       (3) Arthritis of the joints.
    d. Diagnosis is almost always made from culture of the original infection site. Cultures of the blood, joint aspirate, and skin lesions are often negative.

C. Residual of GC PID
1. Narrowing and thickening of the tubes—adnexa are palpable and fixed. May lead to sterility or increases incidence of ectopic pregnancy.
2. Closure of the tubes, usually at fimbriated end, resulting in sterility
3. Pelvic masses secondary to adhesions
4. Uterus fixed and nonmobile secondary to adhesions.
5. May have chronic pain, abnormal uterine bleeding, and/or dyspareunia

D. Effects in pregnancy
1. GC PID during pregnancy can be of greater clinical severity than in nonpregnant women due to suppression of the immune response during pregnancy.
2. There is a greater risk of disseminated GC in pregnant women than in nonpregnant women.
3. Associated with chorioamnionitis, premature rupture of membranes, and premature delivery
4. After delivery, the GC that were present in the vagina can ascend and cause postpartum endometritis.

E. Effects on the fetus and neonate
1. Increased fetal loss and low birth weight if the mother is infected during pregnancy

2. GC infects the infant's conjunctivae as it passes through the vagina during birth, and can cause blindness.
3. The infant can contract disseminated GC.

IV. **Differential Diagnosis**
   A. Depending on site of GC infection
      1. Urethra: Rule out UTI, chlamydia.
      2. Cervix, vagina, Bartholin's: Rule out nongonococcal infection, particularly chlamydia.
      3. Endometrium and/or endosalpinx, Rule out:
         a. Round ligament pain
         b. Diverticulitis
         c. Appendicitis
         d. Ectopic pregnancy
         e. Septic abortion
         f. Pelvic endometriosis
         g. Kidney stone

V. **Management**
   A. Diagnosis is by GC culture of the cervix or urethra if signs and symptoms of urethritis.
   B. Do a GC culture of the cervix at the following times:
      1. Signs and symptoms of gonorrhea
      2. The patient is diagnosed as having syphilis or chlamydia.
      3. The patient expresses a concern that she may have a sexually transmitted infection (STI).
   C. If the culture is positive:
      1. Obtain a venereal disease research laboratory (VDRL), to rule out syphilis before treatment.
      2. The patient may be treated in the office. The Health Department needs to be notified of infection and treatment.
   D. Standard treatment recommended by Centers for Disease Control:
      1. Nonpregnant
         a. Rocephin 250 mg IM one time, followed by doxycyline 100 mg orally twice a day for 7 days
         b. Alternate regimens
            (1) Spectinomycin 2 g IM one time, followed by Doxycycline
            (2) If infection was acquired from a source not proven to be penicillin-resistant, can give amoxicillin 3 g orally with 1 g probenecid followed by doxycycline.
      2. Pregnant
         a. Rocephin 250 mg IM one time plus Erythromycin 500 mg orally four times a day for 7 days
         b. Alternative regime: Spectinomycin 2 g IM followed by Erythromycin
   E. After treatment follow up as below:

1. Reculture cervix after treatment at the following times. If results positive at any time, retreat.
    a. One week after treatment is completed
    b. If gonorrhea diagnosed during pregnancy
        (1) Reculture cervix within 1 month of EDC to verify cure and/or rule out reinfection before delivery.
        (2) Reculture cervix at 6 weeks postpartum visit.
2. The patient should be told of her diagnosis, educated about GC, and the necessity of completion of treatment and follow up.
3. Every effort should be made to contact the patient's sexual partner(s) and confirm their treatment through the Health Department.

F. If gonorrhea was diagnosed during pregnancy
1. Be sure the pediatrician or neonatal nurse practitioner is notified of the fact after delivery.
2. Be alert for signs of GC PID in the postpartum patient and consult with physician if it develops.

NOTES

GRAND MULTIPARITY

I. **Definition:** A grand multipara is a woman who has given birth to five or more children.
II. **Clinical Features**
   A. Potential antepartum complication
      1. Anemia, especially if pregnancies spaced less than a year apart
      2. Obesity
      3. Hypertension
      4. Placenta previa
   B. Intrapartum and postpartum
      1. Abnormal presentation
      2. Precipitous labor, delivery, or both
      3. Dystocias of labor due to poor muscle tone
      4. Large-for-gestation-age infant with attendant problems at delivery (eg, shoulder dystocia)
      5. Postpartum hemorrhage
III. **Management**
   A. At the initial visit, ascertain gravidity and parity. Ask specifically whether any of the complications in section II above were present with previous pregnancies.
   B. Usual management plan
      1. Antepartum
         a. Be alert for potential problems.
         b. Plan for birth in hospital, not birth center.
         c. If previous history of large babies, plan delivery at term to avoid macrosomia.
         d. If previous history of precipitous labor and/or delivery:
            (1) Instruct patient/couple to go to the hospital at the first sign of labor.
            (2) Instruct patient/couple in emergency childbirth management.
         e. Discuss family planning with patient/couple.
      2. Intrapartum
         a. Be sure on-call physician is notified of patient's admission to the hospital.
         b. Prophylactic IV or heparin lock recommended
      3. Postpartum: Be alert for potential postpartum hemorrhage in first 24 hours. Consider prophylactic oxytocin IV immediately after delivery of the placenta.

HEADACHE

I. **Definition:** Diffuse pain in various parts of the head.
II. **Etiology and Management**
   A. Evaluate site, frequency, severity, predisposing factors, etc.
   B. Recommend treatment based on etiology.
   1. Estrogen and progesterone headaches:
      a. Etiology: Occur in early pregnancy, due to hormonal changes, increased cerebral swelling, increased estrogen levels. The typical estrogen headache:
         (1) Occurs in the morning
         (2) Is frontal in distribution
         (3) Is steady
      b. Treatment
         (1) Tylenol, one to two tablets orally every 4 hours as needed
         (2) If Tylenol does not relieve, Fioricet or compounds with codeine, such as Tylenol #3, may be used.
   2. Hypoglycemia—treatment:
      a. Small frequent meals at least every 3 hours
      b. Avoid long periods without food.
      c. Have some protein food at each snack or meal.
      d. Avoid sugars and highly refined foods
      e. May require referral to dietitian
   3. Sinus congestion
   4. Eye strain—treatment:
      a. Instruct regarding proper lighting, reduce glare, etc.
      b. Ascertain whether patient is reading or doing other fine eye work for long periods of time.
      c. May need eye examination
   5. Pre-eclampsia, high blood pressure:
      a. Seen most often in last trimester
      b. Treatment—see Hypertension on page 163.
   6. Tension/Fatigue—treatment:
      a. Investigate cause, reduce or eliminate.
      b. Frequent rest periods
      c. Neck massage, progressive relaxation
      d. May need appropriate referral: Physical therapy, mental health counseling, etc.
   7. Anemia
      a. Usually occur in the afternoon
      b. Treatment—see Anemia on page 72.
   8. Migraine:

a. Usually unilateral and throbbing, accompanied by light flashes, visual disturbances
b. Treatment
    (1) Elicit family history or previous personal history of migraines.
    (2) **Do not** use ergot-based medications, which are commonly used for migraines but are dangerous in pregnancy because of their oxytocic properties.

NOTES

HELLP SYNDROME

I. **Definition:** A syndrome in pregnancy that includes hypertension with hemolysis, elevated liver enzymes and low platelets.
II. **Etiology:** Arteriolar vasospasm is considered the underlying factor. Lesions develop in the endothelial layer of the small blood vessels as a result of vasospasm. Platelets aggregate at the site of the lesion. Red blood cells are forced through the sieve-like structure due to increased pressure, resulting in red blood cell fragments and hyperbilirubinemia. Thrombocytopenia is seen as platelets are consumed in the microcirculation.
III. **Clinical Features**
   A. Arteriolar vasospasm
      1. Decreased cerebral blood flow
         a. Headaches
         b. Scotoma
      2. Hypertension
      3. Decreased uterine blood flow
         a. Intrauterine fetal growth retardation (IUFGR)
         b. Intrapartum fetal hypoxia
         c. Fetal demise
   B. Endothelial damage
      1. Microangiopathic hemolytic anemia
         a. Platelet consumption
         b. Thrombocytopenia
      2. Red cell destruction
         a. Decreased Hct
         b. Hyperbilirubinemia
      3. Glomerular damage
         a. Proteinuria
         b. Oliguria: increased blood urea nitrogen and creatinine
      4. Hepatic congestion
         a. Right upper quadrant pain
         b. Increased serum glutamic-oxaloacetic transaminase (SGOT), decreased serum glutamic-pyruvic transaminase (SGPT)
         c. Decreased blood glucose
   C. Incidence: Occurs in 4% to 12% of severe pre-eclamptic and/or eclamptic patients and is associated with poor maternal and fetal outcome.
   D. Signs and symptoms
      1. Hypertension
      2. Edema
      3. Proteinuria
      4. Fatigue

5. Nausea, vomiting. or both
6. Epigastric or right upper quadrant pain
E. Labwork
   1. CBC with platelet count. Decreased hematocrit and thrombocytopenia are diagnostic.
   2. SMAC-20, lab values will show hyperbilirubinemia, increased SGOT, increased blood urea nitrogen and creatinine and a decreased blood glucose.
   3. Urine dip and catheterized specimen will reveal proteinuria, 24-hour urine will have excessive protein.
F. Management
   1. Refer to physician.
   2. Conservative approach is contraindicated in a patient with HELLP; she must be delivered expeditiously to prevent potentially irreversible complications for the mother or fetal demise.

NOTES

HEMORRHOIDS

I. **Definition:** Anal varicosities.
II. **Etiology**
   A. Genetic predisposition
   B. During pregnancy:
      1. Increased venous pressure on the pelvic veins due to the pressure of the enlarging uterus
      2. The relaxing effect of progesterone on the vein walls and valves, surrounding muscle tissue and large bowel
      3. Trauma from pushing during the second stage of labor and pressure of the baby and distention at birth
III. **Management**
   A. Examine for severity, trauma, and possible thrombosis.
   B. If thrombosed, refer to surgeon or gastrointestinal (GI) specialist for lancing.
   C. Begin comfort measures/medications listed below. If no improvement after 1 week, re-examine. Rule out rectal fissures.
   D. If bleeding continues over 1 month, refer to GI specialist.
   E. Comfort measures
      1. Review diet and modify to keep stools soft.
      2. Relieve constipation.
      3. Take frequent sitz baths. The heat of the water not only gives comfort, but also increases circulation.
      4. Ice packs for reduction of swelling
      5. Rubber ring to sit on can reduce pressure on hemorrhoids and will not interfere with circulation if it is:
         a. Not fully inflated, but inflated only enough to relieve pressure
         b. Large enough to avoid a small area of concentrated pressure
         c. Positioned so that there are no pressure points in the pelvic area
      6. Keep reduced by gently pushing hemorrhoids inside rectum with a lubricated finger cot or glove, then tightening the rectal sphincter to give them support and to contain them within the rectum.
      7. Bedrest with hips and lower extremities elevated
   F. Medications
      1. Colace 50 mg orally every day or twice a day
      2. Preparation H, Proctofoam HC
      3. Suppositories as needed: Anusol, one twice a day and after bowel movement
      4. Tucks (witch hazel packs) to reduce swelling and ease pain
      5. Epsom salt compresses for reduction of swelling
      6. Topical analgesic/anesthetic spray or ointment Americaine Spray, dibucaine ointment.
      7. If bleeding, consider suppositories with cortisone.

HEPATITIS

I. **Definition:** Inflammation of the liver
II. **Etiology**
   A. Type A: Spread predominantly by oral-fecal route
      1. Usually associated with:
         a. Overcrowding
         b. Poor hygiene
         c. Breakdown in normal sanitary conditions (eg, contaminated food or water)
      2. Those at risk:
         a. Institutionalized persons
         b. Children in day care centers
         c. Male homosexuals
         d. IV drug users
         e. Travelers to endemic areas
         f. Military personnel
   B. Type B
      1. Spread predominantly by the parenteral route. Those at risk are those exposed to blood and needles.
         a. Blood transfusions recipients
         b. IV drug users
         c. Medical personnel
         d. Dialysis patients
      2. Found in saliva, semen, and other biological fluids. Cases are associated with close contact with an infected person.
         a. Spouses and other sexual contacts
         b. Male homosexuals
         c. Children of an infected person
   C. Type C: Routes of transmission are the same as type B.
   D. Other causes of acute hepatitis
      1. Mononucleosis, cytomegalovirus
      2. Syphilis
      3. Cholangitis, especially gallstone obstruction
      4. Drug-induced hepatitis: Many medications can cause acute liver injury. Most common are:
         a. Aspirin in high doses
         b. Acetaminophen in high does
         c. Nitrofurantoin
         d. Sulfonamide
   E. Comparison of hepatitis types A, B, and C (see Table 3-2).

Table 3-2. Comparison of Hepatitis Types A, B, and C

Characteristic	A	B	C
Incubation period	14–15 d	40–180 d	15–300 d
Spread	Fecal-oral	Parenteral	Parenteral
blood	No	Yes	Yes
feces	Yes	No	Yes
saliva	Yes	Yes	?
perinatal	No	Yes	?
heterosexual	?	Common	Common
homosexual	Common	Common	Common
male	35%	60%	5%
Immune globulin	Immune globulin	Immune globulin, hepatitis B immune globulin	None
Vaccine	None	Heptavax	Alpha interferon 3 million units 3 × wk × 6 mo

1. Hepatitis D (Delta Agent)—This delta agent is a defective viral agent RNA genome identified only with hepatitis B in the presence of hepatitis B surface antigen (Hb_sAg). When present, the infection is more severe.
2. Hepatitis E—An enterically transmitted form seen in Asia and North Africa

III. **Clinical Features**
   A. Extremely variable—can be:
      1. Mild, transient, and/or asymptomatic.
      2. Severe, prolonged, and/or ultimately fatal.
      3. Anywhere in between
   B. Separated into four phases:
      1. Incubation phase
      2. Pre-icteric phase
      3. Icteric phase
      4. Convalescence
   C. Symptoms according to phase
      1. Incubation period: None
      2. Pre-icteric phase (2–15 days):
         a. Malaise is most frequent complaint; it is the first symptom to appear and the last to resolve.
         b. Anorexia: May have intolerance for strong odors and tastes
         c. Weight loss of 2 to 10 pounds

d. Intermittent nausea and vomiting; may be provoked by eating or smelling food.
e. Distaste for cigarettes in smokers.
f. Right upper quadrant pain: dull, mild to moderate in severity.
g. Less common symptoms
   (1) Low-grade fever
   (2) Headaches
   (3) Diarrhea
3. Icteric phase:
   a. Jaundice is maximal in 1 to 2 weeks and lasts for 6 to 8 weeks.
   b. Pruritus secondary to jaundice
   c. Darkening of urine color
   d. Lightening of stool color
4. Convalescent phase
   a. Begins with disappearance of jaundice and major symptoms and lasts 2 to 6 weeks
   b. Malaise may persist for weeks or months.

D. Signs
1. Mild to moderate hepatic tenderness to percussion
2. Firm liver edge palpable slightly below right costal margin
3. Enlarged spleen may be palpable.
4. Skin manifestation
   a. Rash in 10% to 15% in pre-icteric phase
   b. Excoriations secondary to pruritus
5. Signs of portal hypertension, cirrhosis, hepatic failure

IV. **Maternal, Fetal, and Neonatal Considerations**
A. Maternal considerations
   1. Maternal disease may cause an increase in spontaneous abortion and prematurity.
   2. Maternal disease may possibly be increased in severity in third trimester due to the added load on the liver from the pregnancy.
   3. Preventing maternal hepatitis
      a. Immune globulin may be given if the woman is exposed to hepatitis.
         (1) Give IG for type A.
         (2) Give hepatitis B immune globulin for type B.
      b. Hepatitis B vaccine (Heptavax) may be given to those who are at high risk for contracting hepatitis B. It consists of killed virus, which should be safe in pregnancy, but which has not been widely tested.
B. Fetal considerations
   1. Maternal disease may cause an increase in spontaneous abortion and prematurity.

2. There may be congenital effects from maternal type B infection, irrespective of time of gestation, but it is rare.
3. The major effects on the fetus are secondary to the mother's condition, which may be compromised by the disease, for example, poor nutrition, weight loss, etc. The prognosis is good if the mother has good supportive care.

C. Neonatal considerations
1. The infant may contract the infection in utero or from the mother after birth. Prophylaxis:
   a. Type A: Infants born to mothers who are incubating the virus or are acutely ill should receive one dose of 0.5 ml IG as soon as possible after birth.
   b. Type B: Infants born to Hb_sAg-positive mothers should receive 0.5 hepatitis B immune globulin as soon as possible after birth and 3 and 6 months later. Prophylactic Heptavax given to newborns may offer protection in later life.
   c. Type C: None
2. Virus is shed in the breastmilk, so breastfeeding is contraindicated if the mother is infected.

V. Management

A. At the initial visit ask:
   1. If the patient has ever had blood transfusion. If so, did she have any unusual or abnormal reaction.
   2. If she or anyone in her family has ever had hepatitis.
B. A hepatitis B screen should be ordered on all OB patients.
C. A total hepatitis A, B, and C screen including antigens and antibodies should be ordered on the following:
   1. Those with a positive history of:
      a. Blood transfusion or hepatitis of self or family member
      b. Being rejected as a blood donor because found to be Hb_sAg-positive
      c. Being identified as a carrier
   2. Those with high exposure
      a. Who work or reside in institutions for the mentally retarded, military, day care
      b. Who are exposed to blood and needles
      c. Who have family members who have hepatitis or are carriers
   3. Those from high-risk areas such as Asia, Africa, Pacific Islands
D. A hepatitis screen should be ordered for any client who presents with a clinical picture of hepatitis.
E. If the hepatitis screen is abnormal at any time, order liver function tests. Impaired liver function and/or active infection are indications for physician referral.
F. Any diagnosis of hepatitis must be reported to the Health Department for epidemiologic follow-up.

- **G.** Consider giving vaccine or immune globulin under appropriate conditions.
    1. Exposure to disease, for example, a needle stick with a contaminated needle or contact with a diagnosed person:
        - **a.** Immune globulin (or hepatitis B immune globulin) is most appropriate to prevent contracting the disease.
        - **b.** May offer vaccine later if risk of exposure remains high.
    2. Plans to travel where hepatitis is endemic: Immune globulin is most appropriate because greatest risk to traveler is type A, for which there is no vaccine.
- **H.** Collaborative management is possible for uncompromised, nonacute patients.

NOTES

HERPES SIMPLEX

I. **Definition:** A vesicular eruption of the skin and mucous membranes caused by the herpes virus

II. **Etiology**

   A. There are two types of herpes virus, which have crossreacting antibodies.

   1. Type I is almost always nongenital. The primary infection usually occurs in infancy through prepuberty.
   2. Type II is almost always genital. The primary infection usually occurs after puberty in the sexually active years.
   3. There is some crossover. About 15% of type I herpes is genital and 15% of type II herpes is oral.

   B. Unlike most viruses, the herpes virus does not undergo immune elimination. Despite the presence of specific antibodies, it persists as a latent virus in humans. Recurrences of herpes virus can be triggered by:

   1. Illness
   2. Emotional stress
   3. Intense sunlight
   4. Genital irritation (eg, intercourse or chafing)
   5. Menstruation
   6. Poor nutrition

   C. See Table 3-3 for a comparison of the primary versus recurrent signs and symptoms.

III. **Clinical Features**

   A. Course of illness

   1. Incubation period is 2 to 20 days, averaging 6 days.
   2. Each outbreak consists of three stages:

      a. Prodromal stage: Person feels a vague sensation at the site of viral entry. Sensations include:

         (1) Feeling of pressure
         (2) Dull, pulse-like throbbing
         (3) Intermittent prickly pain
         (4) Tingly sensation
         (5) Ache or soreness at site

      b. Vesicle stage: Red painful vesicular lesions appear that are 1 to 5 mm in diameter, in close proximity to each other, and become confluent.

         (1) In primary episodes, lesions tend to be larger and cover a larger area. In recurrent episodes, lesions are fewer in number, smaller, and usually appear only at the viral entry site.
         (2) In primary episodes, lack of immediate cell-mediated immunity commonly causes systemic signs and symptoms.

Table 3-3. Comparison of Signs and Symptoms of Primary Versus Recurrent Herpes

Signs/Symptoms	Primary	Recurrent
Ulcerated lesions	Multiple	Scattered, 1–3
Location of lesions	Anywhere in genital region, mutiple locations	Confined to one specific area
Size of lesions	Variable, some large	Tend to be smaller than in primary herpes
Duration of lesions	14–28 d	5–10 d
Inguinal adenopathy	Present	Absent
Viremia	Occurs	Absent
Systemic signs: malaise, myalgia headache, fever	Occur if no antibodies to other type	Absent
Local signs: pain, vaginal discharge, dysuria, itching, dyspareunia	Present	Present, also may get prodromal feeling before lesions appear
Specific antibody titer	>Fourfold >Between initial lesion and 1–2 wks later	No significant change

        (a) Chills and fever
        (b) Headache
        (c) Myalgia
        (d) Immune adenopathy
        (e) Crusting-over stage: After 2 to 3 days, the vesicles rupture, leaving painful shallow ulcers with a pale yellow center and bright red border, which persist about a week and then heal without scarring.
  B. Clinical features of oral herpes
    1. Vesicular eruption of gingiva, buccal mucosa, tongue, and soft palate
    2. Yellow-gray membrane forms and sloughs, leaving ulcer
    3. Usually enlarged, tender submandibular lymph nodes
    4. May last 1 to 3 weeks
  C. Clinical features of genital herpes
  D. Diagnosis
    1. Culture
      a. Most accurate test takes 3 to 7 days before results known
      b. To obtain:
        (1) If roofed vesicle:
          (a) Unroof with sterile needle.

(b) Absorb fluid with sterile cotton applicator.
(c) Inoculate medium.
(2) If ulcerated, swab with cotton applicator presoaked in transport medium.
(3) If no lesions, but testing for virus shedding:
(a) Swab cervical canal and site of previous lesion.
(b) Inoculate medium.
(4) All swabs obtained at a single collecting session may go into a single vial, unless it is necessary to localize the site of viral shedding.

2. Blood antibody titers
   a. Obtain at time of initial lesion and repeat in 7 to 10 days if necessary.
   b. Results
      (1) If primary infection:
         (a) No antibodies in blood when tested at time of initial lesion appearance unless person has had herpes elsewhere and has crossreacting antibodies.
         (b) Antibodies appear 7 to 14 days after first sign of infection and reach maximum increase of fourfold or greater within several weeks.
         (c) Thereafter, titers fall to baseline and stay there for life.
      (1) If recurrent infection:
         (a) Antibodies are present in blood when drawn at time of appearance of lesion.
         (b) Blood titer does not rise fourfold as in primary infection.

IV. Management
A. At initial visit, ask about history of herpes.
   1. Patients at risk in pregnancy include:
      a. History of diagnosed genital herpes
      b. History of recurrent vascular or painful genital lesions
      c. Partner with herpes. If the partner has herpes and the patient does not, suggest use of condoms during pregnancy and avoid intercourse from time of partner's prodromal feeling until all lesions are gone.
   2. If definite or probable history of herpes:
      a. Educate patient regarding risks during pregnancy and at time of delivery.
      b. Instruct patient to call you if any outbreaks occur.
      c. Educate regarding palliative measures.
   3. Note history of herpes in chart.
B. Physical exam
   1. If lesions suggestive of herpes are seen:
      a. Perform herpes culture.

b. Ascertain whether primary or secondary infection.
      (1) Previous history of genital lesions
      (2) Recent exposure
      (3) Clinical symptoms. such as malaise, fever, headache
      (4) If primary outbreak, do antibody titers.
   c. Educate regarding palliative measures.
   2. If Pap smear suggestive of herpes is obtained, do herpes culture of any lesions present, or if no lesions, do herpes culture of cervix.
C. If lesions suggestive of herpes appear at any time during the pregnancy, instruct the patient to come in for a culture as soon as possible after lesions appear
D. Management of pregnant patients known to have had genital herpes:
   1. Check patient every week after 36 weeks' EGA for lesions.
   2. If lesion is present:
      a. Culture and follow closely for signs and symptoms of labor.
      b. Sore must be healed approximately 7 days before attempting a vaginal birth, otherwise a cesarean section needs to be scheduled.
E. Medications
   1. Acyclovir is a drug that reduces the severity, duration, and length of viral shedding. It is not recommended for pregnant or lactating patients. It may be prescribed for patients as follows:
      a. Zovirax (acyclovir) ointment 5% to all lesions every 3 to 4 hours until lesions are gone.
      b. Zovirax 200 mg orally every 4 hours while awake or 400 mg twice a day for 7 to 10 days at the first sign of an outbreak.
      c. For frequent outbreaks with lesions every 4 to 6 weeks, consider suppressive management, Zovirax 400 mg orally twice a day or 800 mg every day.
   2. Valtrex (valacyclovir) 500 mg orally twice a day for 5 to 7 days.
   3. Famvir (famciclovir) 125 mg orally twice a day for 5 to 7 days.
F. Comfort
   1. Urinating in sitz bath or while pouring warm over the vulva may reduce pain from urine passing over lesions.
   2. Sitz baths for 15 to 20 minutes three times a day in warm or cool water reduces discharge, odor, and discomfort. May add Burow's solution (aluminum acetate) to the water to help dry out the infected area.
   3. Dry vulva and perineum after sitz bath with a blow dryer on lowest setting.
   4. Do not use creams, ointments, or salves on lesions. They cut off lesions from drying effect of air and light, and could spread virus to a larger area. An exception is Zovirax (Acyclovir) ointment, which may help control the lesions.
   5. Warm damp tea bags (of black tea) are soothing and drying on active lesions.

6. Wear cotton underwear to aid drying; change frequently.
7. Avoid use of restrictive, chafing clothing and pantyhose.
8. OTC pain medications
9. L-Lysine supplements 2 g daily may help heal and prevent future outbreaks.

G. Support measures—refer to herpes support group.

V. **Fetal and Neonatal Considerations**
   A. Congenital problems
      1. First trimester
         a. Increase of spontaneous abortion with primary infection
         b. If the fetus survives, it may have congenital anomalies similar to those caused by cytomegalovirus
      2. Second and third trimesters
         a. There is an increased rate of premature birth if the mother has a primary infection after 20 weeks' gestation.
         b. Infections are associated with low birth weight.
   B. Neonatal infection
      1. Etiology
         a. Usually caused by passing through infected birth canal
         b. Can be contracted from being handled by infected people
      2. Incidence: If the mother had a primary case of genital herpes at term and the birth is vaginal, there is a 50% chance that the infant will have a clinically apparent infection. The incidence drops to less than 3% if the mother has a recurrent case of active herpes at delivery.
      3. Signs and symptoms will appear 4 to 10 days after delivery. Some infected neonates have cutaneous lesions. Other signs and symptoms may include, lethargy, high or low temperature, anorexia, nausea and vomiting, cough or respiratory distress, and irritability or convulsions.

HUMAN IMMUNODEFICIENCY VIRAL DISEASE (HIV)

I. **Definition:** A disease that compromises the competency of the immune system and that is characterized by opportunistic infections

II. **Etiology:** It is caused by the human immunodeficiency virus (HIV) transmitted by exchange of body fluids (ie, semen, blood, saliva) or by transfused blood products. The indicator of the immunodeficiency is depletion of T4+ helper lymphocytes, primarily the result of the attraction of the virus for these lymphocytes.

III. **Clinical Features**
   A. History—comprehensive with special attention to the following:
      1. Current/most recent sexual activity
      2. Type of sexual activity
      3. Use of contraception
      4. Knowledge of preventive measures
      5. Support system and resources
         a. Financial
         b. Emotional
         c. Social
      6. Knowledge of HIV, routes of transmission
      7. History of sexual abuse/physical abuse
   B. Review for signs and symptoms
      1. Fatigue, malaise
      2. Fever, night sweats
      3. Dermatologic lesions, flaking
      4. Lymphadenopathy
      5. Diarrhea
      6. Oral/gingival changes, thrush
      7. Dysphagia
   C. Laboratory
      1. Screen with an enzyme-linked immunoadsorbent assay.
      2. If positive, confirm with the Western blot assay.

III. **Management**
   A. Antepartum: Patients who test positive for acquired immunodeficiency syndrome (AIDS) but do not have acute disease may be collaboratively managed. When managing these patients consider:
      1. Performing a complete exam for HIV progression every trimester
      2. Repeat labs every trimester
         a. CD4
         b. CBC
         c. Syphilis screening
         d. Hbsa
         e. Hepatitis A antibody

- f. Hepatitis C antibody
- g. Gonorrhea culture
- h. Chlamydia testing
- I. Toxoplasmosis
- j. Cytomegalovirus
- k. Chemistry panel
3. Fetal assessment: routine OB plus ultrasound at 16, 28, and 36 weeks' EGA and NST starting weekly at 32 weeks' EGA
4. Social support: Peer group, buddy system, social service as necessary
5. Psychological, substance abuse intervention as necessary
6. Referral to nutritionist
7. Drug therapy: Consult with physician. Usually:
    - a. Start on AZT when the CD4 count is less than 500
    - b. CBC at initiation of AZT, 2 weeks after first dose and monthly to assess bone marrow suppression
    - c. Studies have indicated that giving AZT in the antepartum period will decrease the incidence of HIV transmission to babies of infected patients.

B. Intrapartum
1. Universal precautions
2. Avoid interrupting fetal scalp integrity with scalp electrode.
3. Caesarean section for standard indications
4. Drain umbilical cord for cord blood. Do not use a needle.
5. Collect requested and consented study samples.
6. Use wall rather than mouth suction for DeLee traps.

C. Postpartum
1. Referral for ongoing medical care
2. Referral for baby care
3. Contraception
4. Safe sex counseling
5. Hepatitis vaccine if not given prenatally
6. Pneumococcal vaccine if not given prenatally
7. Rubella vaccine if indicated
8. Social service, psychological, psychiatric, substance abuse counseling follow-up as needed.

HUMAN PAPILLOMA VIRUS/CONDYLOMATA ACUMINATA

I. **Definition:** Genital warts caused by HPV.

II. **Etiology**

A. Caused by HPV, most commonly types 6, 11, 16, 18, 31, or combinations of these.

B. Sexually transmitted

C. Moderate infectivity

D. Multiplies profusely when the immune response is lowered, for example, in HIV, pregnancy, smoking, malnutrition

III. **Clinical Features**

A. Incubation period is from 2 to 3 weeks to 7 to 9 months after exposure but could be longer.

B. May appear on the vulva, vagina, anus, or cervix; the penis and anal area in men.

C. Wart-like growths that are small, discrete structures that spread, enlarge and coalesce to form narrow-based pedunculated cauliflower growths. May appear in one small clump or in many clumps of varying size.

D. Lesions hypertrophy during pregnancy and may cover the vulva and perineum, and/or extend over the vaginal mucosa and cervix. They regress after delivery.

E. Because warts have been linked to the development of cancer, any patient with atypical or persistent warts (and all cervical warts) should have a Pap smear, colposcopy/biopsy, and be treated.

IV. **Differential Diagnosis**

A. Do not confuse with condylomata lata, which are highly infectious secondary syphilitic lesions caused by the spirochete *Treponema pallidum* (See Syphilis on page 232).

B. Comparison of the two

1. Lata appears on the external genitalia only; HPV warts appear in the vagina and on the cervix.

2. Lata looks like a grouping of small, flat warts covered with a grayish exudate.

3. Lata appears only as the primary lesion of syphilis; HPV may appear any time, but proliferates greatly during pregnancy.

4. *Treponema pallidum* can be cultured from lata; HPV from genital warts.

V. **Management**

A. General management, whether pregnant or not

1. Perform a Pap smear for any atypical or persistent warts, and all cervical warts.

2. Patients with external genital warts need a colposcopy. Fifty to sixty percent of clients with external warts will test positive for HPV on the cervix.

3. Identify and treat any accompanying vaginitis to decrease abnormal vaginal secretions.
4. Bichloracetic or trichloracetic acid therapy
   a. The day before treatment have patient sit for 15 minutes in Instant Ocean Salt twice.
   b. Protect the surrounding tissue with petroleum jelly.
   c. Apply bichloroacetic acid (BCA) or trichloroacetic acid (TCA) to affected area every week. Continue as long as warts are regressing. Alternative method is to order Condylox self-treatment kit for the patient.
   d. If no improvement after 4 weeks, consider alternate therapy including cryosurgery, laser, or excision biopsy.
5. For pain relief:
   a. Warm or cool sitz baths as needed
   b. Tylenol regular or extra strength every 4 hours as needed
   c. Nupercainal ointment
6. Advise patient to keep vulva as clean and dry as possible.
   a. Frequent perineal hygiene
   b. Dry after washing or sitz bath with blow dryer set on lowest setting.
   c. Wear cotton underwear, change frequently.
7. Advise couple to use condoms until all lesions are resolved.
8. Consider the possibility of coexisting STDs.

B. Additional management specific to the pregnant patient
   1. Avoid episiotomy or laceration through lesions at time of delivery because they bleed profusely.
   2. An episiotomy at an odd angle to avoid the lesions may be indicated.
   3. For extensive lesions, consult with physician. Caesarean section may be indicated.

C. For management of cervical lesions, see section on Cervical Abnormalities on page 94.

HYDATIDIFORM MOLE

I. **Definition:** A developmental tumor of the placenta, originating in the trophoblastic cells that develop into the placenta. The trophoblastic cells are fast-growing and invasive, like cancer. It is believed that most spontaneously abort in the first trimester.

II. **Incidence**
   A. Occurs in 1 in 200 pregnancies in the United States
   B. Recurs in 2% of women who have had them
   C. Women over 45 have a 10 times greater incidence.
   D. Two to eight percent of molar pregnancies are malignant.

III. **Clinical Features**
   A. Signs and symptoms
      1. Can appear to be a normal pregnancy
      2. Great increase in human chorionic gonadotropin (hCG) levels due to rapid proliferation of placental cells, which excrete hCG
      3. Hyperemesis gravidarum in 30% of these patients because the increased placental tissue overstimulates the corpus luteum and there is increased hormone production.
      4. Uterus often large for dates because mole grows fast
      5. Often enlarged, tender ovaries.
      6. No FHT
      7. Irregular painless bleeding in most by 12th week. May be continuous or intermittent, usually brownish, not heavy.
      8. Pre-eclampsia before 24 weeks
      9. May be anemic secondary to blood loss and/or poor nutrition due to hyperemesis.
   B. Diagnosis
      1. Can be diagnosed by ultrasound
      2. Passage of pieces of mole—the chorionic villi, which have developed into grape-like vesicles and can break off and be expelled vaginally

IV. **Management**
   A. See section on first-trimester bleeding on page 85.
   B. Refer to physician. Mole needs to be removed.
   C. Hydatidiform mole is usually benign but can become malignant trophoblastic disease.
      1. Types of malignant trophoblastic disease
         a. Choriocarcinoma: Metastasizes quickly early in pregnancy. Fastest growing cancer known; therefore, highly responsive to chemotherapy.
         b. Chorioadenoma: Does not metastasize fast. Curable with hysterectomy if still confined to uterus.
      2. Follow-up treatment of hydatidiform moles after removal:

- a. Monitor serum hCG levels biweekly till negative, then monthly for 1 year. The woman should be encouraged not to become pregnant again until after a year of negative levels.
- b. If patient is Rh(D) negative, she needs RhoGAM.
- c. If malignant, refer for chemotherapy.

NOTES

HYPERTENSION DURING PREGNANCY

I. **Definition**
   A. An increase of 30 mmHg systolic or 15 mmHg diastolic over baseline BP readings.
   B. A BP reading of greater than 140/90
   C. The elevated readings occur on two occasions at least 6 hours apart.

II. **Clinical Features**
   A. Classification
      1. Chronic hypertensive disease: The presence of persistent hypertension, BP greater than 140/90 before pregnancy or before the 20th week of gestation.
      2. Pregnancy-induced hypertension (PIH): The development of hypertension during pregnancy or within the first 24 hours after delivery in a previously normotensive woman. No other evidence of pre-eclampsia or hypertensive vascular disease is seen. The BP goes no higher than 150/100 with activity, rapidly returns to normal with rest, and returns to normotensive levels within 10 days postpartum.
      3. Pre-eclampsia: The development of hypertension with proteinuria, excessive edema, or both. It occurs after 20 weeks' gestation. More common with:
         a. Primigravidas, especially if under 17 or over 35
         b. Family history of pre-eclampsia
         c. Multiple gestation
         d. Hydatidiform mole
      4. Eclampsia: The occurrence of convulsions in a patient with pre-eclampsia.
      5. Superimposed pre-eclampsia or eclampsia: The development of pre-eclampsia or eclampsia in a woman with chronic hypertensive vascular disease or renal disease.
      6. HELLP syndrome (See HELLP Syndrome on page 144.)
   B. Signs and symptoms of pre-eclampsia
      1. Hypertension: Increase of 30 mmHg systolic or 15 mmHg diastolic
      2. Marked hyperreflexia, especially with transient or sustained ankle clonus
      3. Edema of the face
      4. Visual disturbances
      5. Drowsiness or severe headaches (forerunner of convulsion)
      6. A sharp increase in the amount of proteinuria (5 g or more in a 24-hour specimen or 3 to 4+ dipstix)
      7. Oliguria: Urine output less than 30 ml/hr or less than 500 ml/24 hours
      8. Epigastric pain due to liver distention

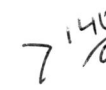

III. **Management**
   A. Initial history
      1. Be alert to any history of:
         a. Previous abruption
         b. Premature labor
         c. IUFGR
         d. Stillbirth
         e. Hypertension when on BCPs
         f. Family history of hypertension
         g. Pre-eclampsia in a previous pregnancy
         h. Previous hypertension, now resolved
      2. Consult with physician if history reveals any of the following:
         a. Two or more consecutive episodes of premature labor, IUFGR, or stillbirth
         b. Chronic hypertension
         c. Severe pre-eclampsia or eclampsia
   B. Prevention
      1. Good prenatal care
         a. Encourage regular visits.
         b. Check weight, BP and urine at each prenatal visit.
      2. Encourage a good diet including:
         a. Adequate weight gain: 20 to 40 pounds
         b. Well-balanced, high-protein diet
   C. Any patient with a questionably elevated BP at prenatal visit should be positioned on her left side for 5 minutes and then the BP retaken before diagnosis is assumed.
   D. If a patient's BP starts rising, institute the following:
      1. Advise rest on the left side 4 to 6 hours a day in addition to her regular night's sleep.
      2. Stop work if still working.
      3. Recommend daily BP checks. If patient, her family, or a friend cannot do, refer for home BP monitoring.
      4. Give fetal movement log and instruct in use.
      5. Schedule for biweekly NST.
      6. Inform of danger signs with instructions to call if any appear:
         a. Headache unrelieved by Tylenol and rest in a dark room
         b. Visual changes
         c. Sudden severe increase in weight and/or edema
         d. Drastic decrease in urine output despite usual intake.
         e. Epigastric pain
      7. Diet counseling.
      8. Increase frequency of office visits; see weekly or biweekly.

E. If hypertension (by definition) develops:
  1. Review history, question regarding presence of any abnormal symptoms.
  2. Conduct physical exam.
     a. Check DTRs for clonus.
     b. Check retinal fundi.
     c. Observe for excessive edema, especially of the hands and face.
  3. Obtain blood workup.
     a. SMAC
        (1) Uric acid—elevated in pre-eclampsia but not in chronic hypertension. Significant if greater than 6.
        (2) Elevated SGOT
     b. CBC
        (1) An elevated Hct may be caused by hemoconcentration
        (2) Platelet count, if low, may indicate vascular damage.
  4. Urine workup
     a. Dipstix of 3⁺ to 4⁺ protein is significant and needs further study.
     b. If catheterized specimen has any protein, further study is required.
     c. Twenty-four-hour urine will test kidney function.
        (1) Total volume should never be less than 500 ml if collected correctly.
        (2) Total protein should not be over 5 g.
        (3) Creatinine, creatinine clearance
  5. Consult with physician to develop a plan of management.
     a. Treatment of choice is delivery if near term.
     b. If patient has seizure:
        (1) Have someone summon physician immediately.
        (2) Protect woman from harming herself.
        (3) Give Valium 10 mg IV slowly (over 1–2 minutes)
        (4) Give $MgSO_4$ 2 g IV push, slowly over 2 to 3 minutes.
        (5) Monitor vital signs immediately after.

INTRAUTERINE FETAL GROWTH RETARDATION (IUFGR)

I. **Definition:** A condition in which a fetus shows clinical evidence of abnormal or dysfunctional growth

II. **Etiology**
   A. Maternal: Alcoholism or drug abuse
   B. Heavy smoking greater than one pack per day
   C. Hypertension or renal disease
   D. Systemic disease, such as cardiac disease
   E. Rubella or other viral infection
   F. History of previous small-for-gestational-age baby
   G. Severe malnutrition
   H. Poor weight gain pattern

III. **Clinical Features**
   A. Types
      1. Symmetric growth retardation—growth is proportional but slow.
      2. Asymmetric—To protect itself, the fetus shunts more food to the brain and other vital organs. The biparietal diameter is at least 2 cm larger than the chest.
   B. Inadequate maternal weight gain—less than 10 pounds in the first half of pregnancy and less than 2 pounds per month in the second half
   C. Size/date discrepancy of concern
      1. If size seemed consistent with dates earlier in the pregnancy and dates are thought to be reliable
      2. If fundal height is 2 cm below the estimated gestational age in weeks
   D. Suspect trisomy 18 if IUFGR is found in first half of pregnancy

IV. **Differential Diagnosis**
   A. Inaccurate fundal measurement
   B. Inaccurate dates
   C. Oligohydramnios (can be diagnosed by ultrasound)
   D. Transverse lie
   E. Small but normal fetus. Suspect this if patient is small-boned, 5 foot tall, with a prepregnant weight of less than 100 pounds.

V. **Management**
   A. If suspect
      1. Will need serial ultrasounds to confirm
      2. If initial ultrasound shows size appropriate for dates and no body/head discrepancy, reassure family that all is within normal limits and no further action is needed.
      3. If initial ultrasound shows size small for dates or other discrepancy, such as mild oligohydramnios or low total intrauterine volume, repeat ultrasound in 1 to 2 weeks.

- **B.** Doppler flow studies can be used to check maternal-fetal-placental unit.
- **C.** If IUFGR is suspected or confirmed by ultrasound, consult with physician. Collaborative management is possible.
- **D.** Management after diagnosis of IUFGR
    1. Treat underlying cause if known.
    2. If patient is a smoker, urge her to quit.
    3. Evaluate diet for adequate protein, calories.
    4. Increase rest, fluids.
    5. Instruct patient to keep daily fetal movement log and call if movements not adequate.
    6. Biweekly nonstress tests with office visits
    7. Obtain fasting blood sugar and 2-hour PP blood sugar to assess carbohydrate metabolism.
    8. May need serial ultrasounds to monitor fetal growth.
    9. Consult with physician regarding the best time to induce this patient. Early delivery is preferred.
    10. Fetal monitor is mandatory in labor.
    11. Notify pediatrician or neonatal nurse practitioner of admission to labor and delivery.

NOTES

ISOIMMUNIZATION

I. **Definition**

   A. Rh isoimmunization is caused by maternal antibody production in response to exposure to fetal RBC antigens of the Rh group, including C, D, and E. The maternal antibody response may cross the placenta, potentially destroying fetal RBCs, causing anemia, and may result in erythroblastosis fetalis.

   B. ABO group O–positive women have anti-A and anti-B isoagglutination, which may cause hemolytic disease in the newborn. Group O–negative women have neither A nor B and their newborns are born without problems.

   C. Over 400 other red cell antigens have been identified. While most have little clinical importance, some are significant and in pregnancy may affect the developing fetus. Some are:

   1. Moderate to severe disease
      a. Kell system: K,k antigens
      b. Duffy system: FY^2 (Fy^b does not cause problems)
      c. Kidd system: Jk^a, Jk^b antigens
   2. Mild hemolytic disease
      a. Kell system: K, Ko, Kpb antigens
      b. Diego system: Di^a, Di^b antigens
      c. MNSs system: M, N antigens
   3. Without problems
      a. Lewis system: All antigens

II. **Incidence**

   A. Rh or D isoimmunization has been reported in 2% of primiparous patients at the time of delivery. Seven percent more will have anti-D 6 months postpartum, and 7% more will go on to develop sensitization in subsequent pregnancies. RhoGAM has reduced these figures when given at the recommended times.

   B. The CDE antigen groupings have racial differences.
   1. Thirteen percent of white Americans are negative.
   2. Seven percent of African Americans are negative.
   3. One percent of Native Americans, those of Chinese descent, and other Asians are negative.

   C. ABO—the mother is O positive, the fetus is A, B, or AB.
   1. Twenty percent of all infants have an ABO incompatibility.
   2. Five percent of newborns will show signs of hemolytic disease.
   3. The later the onset of signs and symptoms, the less severe the problem for the newborn

III. **Clinical Features**

   A. Maternal and fetal blood rarely mix, however, mixing can occur during the following incidents, which can result in sensitization:

1. At time of delivery, especially if accompanied by manual removal of the placenta or other manipulative procedures that result in increased mixing of maternal and fetal blood.
2. During pregnancy, probably due to breaks in the fetal and/or maternal circulation, which result in transfusion of fetal blood to the maternal circulation. It should be suspected if an amniocentesis is performed and in any case of uterine bleeding in pregnancy, such as placenta previa or abruptio placenta.
3. Induced and spontaneous abortions
4. Ectopic pregnancy
5. Trauma

B. If natural antibodies gain access to the fetal circulation, they act as hemolysins to the fetal erythrocytes. Danger to the fetus varies with degree of severity.
 1. In less severe cases, the fetus has jaundice either at birth or soon after due to erythroblastosis with possible resulting kernicterus and/or anemia.
 2. In severe cases, the fetus develops hydrops fetalis, a condition of severe anemia and edema and may die in utero or soon after birth from circulatory collapse and/or anemia and dyspnea.
 3. ABO incompatibility seldom causes hydrops fetalis, but does sometimes cause jaundice.

IV. Management

A. At the initial OB visit, ask about a history of blood transfusions, blood disorders, or problems with previous pregnancies or deliveries, and if the patient is known to be Rh(D) negative. If sensitization is confirmed by antibody titer, refer to perinatologist.

B. Routine labwork
 1. All pregnant patients need to have blood for labwork drawn at the initial visit for D factor and antibody titer.
    a. If the antibody titer is positive, order a repeat titer and an antibody identification. Ask if the patient has recently received a RhoGAM injection because this may cause the titer to be positive. If the problem continues, refer.
    b. If the patient is Rh(D) negative, be sure to counsel her and chart in a prominent place.
 2. A repeat antibody titer should be performed again on all Rh(D)-negative patients between 24 and 28 weeks. Note if the patient has received RhoGAM because of a bleed, amniocentesis, etc. This will cause the titer to convert to a positive.

C. RhoGAM should be administered to all unsensitized Rh(D)-negative patients.
 1. At 28 to 36 weeks gestation
 2. Within 72 hours of the following:
    a. Removal of an ectopic pregnancy
    b. Amniocentesis
    c. Removal of hydatidiform mole

d. An episode of uterine bleeding in pregnancy
   e. Delivery of an Rh(D) positive baby, whether RhoGAM had been given prophylactically at 28 to 30 weeks or not.
3. RhoGAM is passive immunoglobulin that prevents the Rh(D) negative person from producing antibodies against the D antigen, thus preventing sensitization. It is always given intramuscularly.
   a. The standard dose is 1 vial, although micro or macro doses may be given, depending on the amount of mixing of maternal and fetal blood that potentially occurred.
   b. One MICRhoGAM dose appears adequate for abortions up to 12 weeks gestation
   c. One vial Rh(D) immune globulin is adequate to cover up to 15 ml of fetal blood in the maternal circulation.
   d. A Kleinhauer-Betke test may be ordered to determine the amount of fetal blood in the maternal circulation, and thus the dose of RhoGAM needed.
4. RhoGAM should not be administered in the following situations:
   a. Rh(D) positive woman
   b. Sensitized Rh(D) negative woman
   c. Rh(D) negative woman who has given birth to a Rh(D) negative baby
   d. Never give RhoGAM to a baby.

V. **Teaching**
   A. All Rh(D)-negative patients should be counseled regarding the physiology and implications of being Rh(D) negative, and the importance of receiving RhoGAM in situations when sensitization may occur.
   B. After the patient has been given a dose of RhoGAM, be sure the patient is given the lab slip that indicates she has had RhoGAM with the date and dose given.
   C. Patients with other blood group incompatibilities should be counseled/referred as appropriate for that particular antigen.

LUPUS

I. **Definition**
   A. Lupus is a chronic, inflammatory autoimmune disorder in which the body's immune system, instead of serving a normal protective function, forms antibodies that attack healthy tissues and organs.
   B. Types
      1. Discoid lupus erythematosus (DLE) affects the skin, causing a rash, lesions, or both.
      2. Systemic lupus erythematosus (SLE) is usually more severe than DLE. It attacks body organs and systems, such as joints, kidneys, brain, heart, and lungs. It can be life-threatening.
      3. Drug-induced lupus symptoms usually disappear on discontinuance of medication.

II. **Etiology:** Unknown

III. **Clinical Features**
   A. Signs and symptoms
      1. DLE
         a. Exposure to sunlight often precedes the appearance of lesions. Half of patients have a history of photosensitivity.
         b. Lesions are erythematous, round, scaling papules, 5 to 10 mm in diameter, often appearing in a butterfly shape over the bridge of the nose, with some appearing on the trunk, extremities, or both.
         c. The disease is limited to the skin in 90% of DLE patients. Ten percent will go on to develop SLE.
      2. SLE
         a. SLE: Signs and symptoms include the abovementioned rash and are often nonspecific and mimic other diseases.
         b. Frequent UTIs to chronic renal problems
         c. Fever and malaise
         d. Ninety percent have joint pain (Jaccoud's fever)
         e. Recurrent pleurisy
         f. Pericarditis
         g. Hypertension
         h. Splenomegaly
         i. Central nervous system problems: chronic headaches, epilepsy, personality changes to chronic brain syndrome
         j. Depression of hemoglobin, WBCs, platelets
         k. Infertility or increased fetal loss
   B. Laboratory
      1. Skin biopsy studies will not differentiate DLE and SLE, but will rule out other disorders.

2. SLE screening test is the fluorescent test for antinuclear antibodies (ANA). It is positive in 98% of cases. Drugs such as procainamide, hydralazine, and isoniazid will make this test positive.

IV. **Management**
   A. After diagnosis, patient needs to be referred to a specialist.
   B. Patient may be collaboratively managed after initial treatment and plan have been developed.
   C. Considerations in pregnancy
      1. Lupus patients are considered "high risk."
      2. Twenty-five percent of patients have a problem getting pregnant.
      3. Pregnant lupus patients experience frequent miscarriages and still-births.
      4. Thirty-three percent of lupus patients have an antibody that is associated with early failure of the placenta (anti-cardiolipin) and about 10% have a related antibody, lupus anticoagulant, which allows early pregnancy, but, at some point, the baby's growth slows as the placenta fails.
      5. Twenty-five percent of the remaining pregnancies deliver prematurely.
      6. Flare-up of lupus caused by pregnancy sometimes occurs.
         a. Thirty-three percent of patients will have a decrease in platelet count
         b. Twenty percent will have urine protein.
         c. Thirty-three percent will have a sudden increase in blood pressure (pregnancy-induced hypertension) or eclampsia.
      7. Medications while pregnant
         a. Safe: Prednisone, prednisolone, methylprednisolone (Medrol). These do not go through placenta.
         b. Probably safe: Azathioprine and hydroxychloroquine. Consult before giving.
         c. Not recommended unless baby needs treatment as well: dexamethasone and betamethasone
         d. Harmful: cyclophosphamide
   D. Effect on baby
      1. Prematurity is the greatest danger.
      2. There are no known congenital abnormalities peculiar to babies of lupus patients.
      3. Three percent of all lupus patients will have a baby with neonatal lupus. This is a syndrome **not** SLE and is transient. If heart problems occur (rare), they are treatable but permanent.
   E. Family planning considerations
      1. Barrier methods or IUD are best and safest
      2. BCPs might exacerbate lupus but are safer than an unwanted pregnancy.

MAMMOGRAPHY

I. **Definition:** Mammography is the radiographic examination of the breast and is the only reliable means of detecting breast cancer before a mass can be palpated.

II. **Indications**

   A. To evaluate the breast when a diagnosis of potentially curable cancer has been made
   B. To evaluate a questionable breast mass
   C. To screen women who are at risk for developing breast cancer.

III. **Management**

   A. Normal mammogram: follow according to American Cancer Society guidelines:
      1. Baseline mammogram between 35 to 40 years
      2. Mammogram every 2 years after age 40
      3. Mammogram every year after age 50
      4. Mammograms should start at 30 years of age and be done more frequently when there is a family history of breast cancer, fibrocystic breast changes, or breast augmentation.
   B. Abnormal mammogram
      1. Findings suggesting cysts on a mammogram should be sent for breast ultrasound:
         a. If ultrasound confirms simple cyst, it may be drained or followed with mammograms every 6 months.
         b. If ultrasound reveals a noncystic breast problem, refer for needle localization biopsy.
      2. Masses that have a noncystic appearance on mammogram, refer to surgeon.
      3. Microcalcifications: Tiny specks of calcium in the breast are often found in areas of rapidly dividing cells.
         a. Benign appearing: Repeat mammogram in 3 to 6 months.
         b. Clustered or small grouping: Refer for needle localization biopsy and/or removal.
      4. Macrocalcifications: Calcium deposits frequently associated with degenerative changes in the breast due to aging, old injuries, or inflammation.
         a. Usually benign
         b. First appearance: Repeat mammogram in 6 months.
         c. Stable—mammogram every year

MASTITIS

I. **Definition:** Inflammation of the breast
II. **Incidence:** Can occur in anyone but is almost exclusively a complication in the lactating woman
III. **Etiology:** Develops as a result of invasion of breast tissue by bacteria in the presence of breast injury. The most common causative bacterium is *Staphylococcus aureus*.
   A. Causes of injury are:
      1. Bruising from rough manipulation, pumping
      2. Breast overdistention
      3. Milk stasis in a duct
      4. Cracking/fissures of the nipple
   B. Sources from which bacteria may originate:
      1. The hands of the mother
      2. The hands of any person caring for the mother or baby
      3. The baby
IV. **Clinical Features**
   A. Precursory signs and symptoms:
      1. Severe engorgement
      2. Slight fever
      3. Mild pain in one segment of the breast, which is exaggerated when baby nurses
      4. Slight redness over affected area
   B. Mastitis
      1. Rapid elevation in temperature to 100°F to 104°F
      2. Increased pulse rate
      3. Chills, general malaise, headache
      4. Area of breast reddened, very tender, painful with hard sizable lump(s)
      5. C&S done on breast milk may identify the bacteria.
   C. Untreated mastitis may progress to abscess.
      1. Discharge of pus, especially if high temperature continues for more than 48 hours
      2. Remittent fever with chills
      3. Breast swollen and extremely painful; a large, hard mass with an area of fluctuation, reddening, and bluish tinge to the skin, indicating the location of the pus-filled abscess.
IV. **Management**
   A. Treatments of choice are Keflex 500 mg orally four times a day for 7 to 10 days or Augmentin 250 to 500 mg orally three times a day for 7 to 10 days. Advise to take antibiotic for full course even if improved sooner. See in office in 7 to 10 days. May need to retreat.

- **B.** Warn patient that monilia vaginitis may develop secondary to antibiotic therapy. Patient should be alert of signs and symptoms, and may want to use prophylactic vaginal yogurt or acidic tablets while taking antibiotics.
- **C.** Obtain milk C&S from affected breast to confirm diagnosis and treatment as necessary.
- **D.** Advise client to continue breastfeeding unless abscess is present. Hot compress before breastfeeding may be helpful. Continuation of breastfeeding in the presence of abscess is not recommended. Suggest the following:
    1. Discontinue breastfeeding until afebrile for 24 hours, usually about 24 to 48 hours after starting antibiotics, then may resume breastfeeding.
    2. During time breastfeeding is discontinued, pump breasts at least every 4 hours with an electric or manual pump after heat has been applied to the breasts. Avoid manipulation, which will exaggerate the already existing breast injury.
    3. Discard any milk pumped during the time breastfeeding has been discontinued because it may contain pus.
- **E.** Provide firm, nonconstrictive support for the breasts.
- **F.** May require pain medication. If Tylenol is not effective, prescribe Darvon N-100 or Tylenol No. 3.
- **G.** If abscess is present, consult with physician. May need incision and drainage.

NOTES

MENOPAUSE/PERIMENOPAUSE

I. **Definitions**
   A. Menopause is the permanent cessation of menses resulting from ovarian failure.
   B. Perimenopause is the term used to describe the years that surround the actual experience of menopause. This transition usually takes 4 to 5 years and is characterized by menstrual irregularity. Conception is unlikely but can still occur.

II. **Etiology**
   A. Six percent of women enter menopause by 35 years of age; 25% by 44 years of age; 75% by 50 years of age; 94% by 55 years of age.
   B. Estrogen and progesterone levels begin to fluctuate unpredictably.
   C. The cells lining the follicles in the ovary no longer respond as predictably to follicle-stimulating hormone (FSH) or luteinizing hormone (LH), resulting in anovulatory menstrual cycles.
   D. Surgical menopause: Removal of the ovaries and uterus will cause immediate symptoms of change. Removal of only the uterus will allow the ovaries to continue producing estrogen and the signs of change will be more gradual.

III. **Clinical Features**
   A. Change in menstruation
      1. Menstrual cycles:
         a. Often anovulatory
         b. Breakthrough bleeding with spotting days 19 to 25 may occur.
         c. Less frequent periods and skipping of cycles
      2. Amount
         a. Majority experience short, scant bleeding.
         b. Heavier periods with clots and cramps can occur.
   B. Signs and symptoms of premenstrual syndrome (PMS) increase.
      1. Bloating
      2. Pelvic discomfort
      3. Headaches
      4. Irritability
      5. Mood swings
   C. Vasomotor disturbances (hot flashes, night sweats)
      1. Occur in 45% of women
      2. Twenty-five percent have hot flashes for over 5 years.
      3. Two percent experience them for life.
      4. Hot flashes occurring while sleeping cause profuse perspiration.
   D. Urogenital atrophy
      1. Thinner urethral epithelium and less urethral tone may lead to urinary frequency and urgency.
      2. More susceptible to UTIs

3. Loss of support for pelvic viscera
4. Loss of rugation in vagina and paleness of mucosa

E. Osteoporosis
1. Bone is lost at an annual rate of 0.5% after age 40.
2. Common symptoms: height loss, back pain, and increased fractures
3. Most common fractures are vertebral, forearm, and hip.
4. Hip fractures and sequelae are lethal in 12% to 20% of women.

F. Cardiovascular disease
1. Throughout reproductive life, serum levels of low-density lipoprotein (LDL) cholesterol in women are lower than those in men.
2. Levels of LDL cholesterol rise at menopause so they are equal to those of men.
3. No significant change in high-density lipoprotein (HDL) levels
4. Therefore, after menopause, women's risk of cardiovascular disease equals that of men.

G. Skin changes
1. Thinning and loss of subcutaneous fat
2. Dryness
3. Loss of hair
4. Minor hirsutism of face

H. Neuropsychiatric problems
1. Depression and mood changes caused by hormone changes and insomnia are common during the perimenopause.
2. Sexual desire and coital enjoyment decreases in many women.

IV. **Management**
A. History
1. Menstrual history
2. Systems that could be affected by estrogen deficiency
3. Hot flashes
4. Stress incontinence
5. Symptoms and risks for cardiovascular disease
6. Gynecologic surgery?

B. Physical exam should include:
1. Thorough breast exam
2. Inspection of vaginal mucosa for paleness, loss of rugation
3. Careful bimanual exam
   a. In menopause, the ovaries should be very small or not palpable.
   b. The uterus should be small with normal consistency. A firm, irregular, or enlarged uterus may indicate a fibroid or other problems.
4. Inspect for cystocele, rectocele, and uterine prolapse.

5. Rectal exam
C. Laboratory
   1. Pap smear
   2. Mammogram
   3. Blood workup may include:
      a. hCG to determine if pregnant
      b. FSH should be measured on day 6 or 7 of a birth control pill-free week. If above 40 miu/ml, the patient is in menopause and may be switched to, or started on, hormone replacement therapy (HRT).
      c. LH changes little throughout adulthood: female non-midcycle, less than 30 IU/L; midcycle, 30 to 150 IU/L; postmenopausal, 30 to 120 IU/mc. Note: An FSH:LH ratio of greater than one is diagnostic of menopause.
      d. Estradiol (E^2) below 3 ng/dl indicates postmenopausal female.
      e. Progesterone (serum): Measure days 20 to 24 before menses. Patient is anovulatory if below 300 ng.
      f. Thyroid profile may be done to rule out problems in this area.
      g. Prolactin if nipple discharge
      h. Cardiac risk assessment: HDL, LDL, triglycerides
      i. Stool for occult blood
D. Special considerations
   1. Consider endometrial biopsy in the following situations:
      a. Any abnormal uterine bleeding over 35 year of age
      b. Before the initiation of HRT
      c. If a postmenopausal patient presents with vaginal bleeding, a biopsy is a necessity.
   2. If adnexa are found to be young adult size, or enlarged in a menopausal woman, consider ultrasound plus CA 125.
   3. If uterus is firm, enlarged, has an irregular contour, do ultrasound and refer as appropriate.
   4. Urinary incontinence/cystocele
      a. Kegel exercises
      b. If patient is not a good surgical candidate, try a pessary, Introl System.
      c. Refer for workup and probable surgery.
   5. If patient has a family history of osteoporosis or is at high risk by lifestyle, physical characteristics, consider bone density studies.
E. Medications: Perimenopausal
   1. For irregular bleeding without other signs and symptoms:
      a. In a nonsmoker over 35 years of age, try BCPs.
      b. In either smoker or nonsmoker

No estrogen	
Provera 5–10 mg, 1st 10 days of the month	

or

No estrogen	
	Provera 5–10 mg, day 14 or 16 to day 25 of cycle

    2. For irregular bleeding with other signs and symptoms:
        a. In a nonsmoker over 35 years of age

Birth control pills:	Estrogen	Premarin 0.3 mg/day during inert pills
	Progestin	No progestin

        b. In a smoker over 35 years of age: Premphase tablets

Premarin 0.625 daily	
	Provera 5–10 mg, day 14 or 16 to day 25 of cycle

  F. Medications: HRT
    1. Advantages
        a. Relief of menopausal symptoms
        b. Prevention and treatment of osteoporosis
        c. Prevention of cardiovascular disease
    2. Risks
        a. Endometrial cancer: Two to six times greater in women with a uterus using unopposed estrogen
        b. Breast cancer: Slight increased risk of breast cancer with prolonged use of HRT.
    3. Contraindications to HRT
        a. Known breast cancer
        b. Known or suspected endometrial cancer
        c. Known or suspected pregnancy
        d. Undiagnosed genital bleeding
        e. Active thrombophlebitis and thrombotic disorders
        f. Acute liver disease or chronic impaired liver function
    4. Commonly used preparations
        a. Estrogen preparations

- (1) Conjugated estrogens (Premarin, Ogen) 0.625, 1.25 mg
- (2) Micronized estradiol (Estrace) 0.5, 1.0, 2.0 mg
- (3) Estradiol patch (Estraderm, Vivelle, Climara) .05, 0.1 mg
  b. Progestin preparations
     - (1) Medroxyprogesterone acetate (Provera, Cycrin) 2.5, 5, 10 mg
     - (2) Norethindrone .35, 0.7 mg
  c. Estrogen/progestin combined preparations
     - (1) Premarin plus Provera (Prempro) 0.625 mg Premarin plus 2.5 mg Provera
     - (2) Premarin every day plus Provera days 15 to 28 of cycle (Premphase) 0.625 mg Premarin every day with 5 mg of Provera added days 15 to 28
5. Hormone prescribing schedules
   a. Perimenopause regimens: These were designed to mimic Mother Nature. At the end of the progestin administration, vaginal bleeding ensues. These medications do not protect against pregnancy.

Estrogen daily
Provera 5–10 mg, days 1 to 10 every month

Premphase tablets

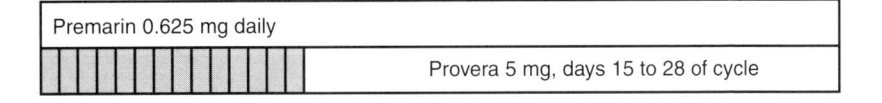

Premarin 0.625 mg daily
Provera 5 mg, days 15 to 28 of cycle

  b. Menopause
     - (1) Continuous-dose regimen leads to further atrophy and thinning of the endometrium. Advantages:
       - (a) If there is still occasional spotting, this combination will ultimately eliminate it.
       - (b) If periods have stopped for mor than 1 year, they are unlikely to restart.

Estrogen daily
Provera 2.5 mg daily

  c. Hysterectomy: Daily estrogen is indicated for women without a uterus. There is no need for progestin administration.

| Estrogen daily |
| No provera |

D. Special problems
1. Unable to take estrogen: Bellergal-S orally twice a day may provide relief from hot flashes.
2. Unable to take Provera due to increased PMS, bloating, gas, and cramps, try Micronor (norethindrone) 0.35 mg/day.
3. If increasing the estrogen dose does not relieve symptoms, try an injectable estrogen every month with or without testosterone (Depo-Estradiol, Depo-Testadiol).
4. Decreased libido: Try Estratest H.S., which has 0.625 of esterified estrogen and 1.25 mg of methyltestosterone. This can be increased to Estratest, which is double strength. An androgen given alone may be used with any combination of estrogen and progesterone to increase sex drive.
5. Atrophic vaginitis, abnormal squamous cells of undetermined significance (ABSCUS) on Pap smear. Ortho Dienestrol, Estrace, Ogen, Premarin, or other vaginal creams can be used locally. When starting estrogen creams, it should be given every day for 1 to 2 weeks, every other day for a week, then two times a week. Some patients can remain symptom-free using estrogen cream once a week.
6. Local irritation at application site with Estraderm and Climara patches. Remove backing, wait 30 to 60 seconds to allow alcohol to evaporate before applying.

V. **Teaching**
A. Instruct regarding signs and symptoms of menopause.
B. Hot flashes can be helped by wearing light clothes, dressing in layers.
C. Insomnia: nap during the day, decrease caffeine and spicy foods, especially at night.
D. Mood swings, irritability, depression can be improved with a regular diet and exercise. Talking with friends helps. If depression is severe (having crying spells, suicidal thoughts), a complete physical and HRT may help. Referral to a counselor or psychologist may be indicated.
E. Exercise should become a way of living and being healthier.
F. Diet low in fat, high in fiber, with calcium-rich foods
G. Diet and supplements must provide 1500 mg calcium per day.
H. For individual problems, such as incontinence, pain with intercourse, heart palpitations, etc., consult with health provider.
I. Take all medication as prescribed. Estrogen, when taken without progesterone, may do more damage than not taking any medicine.

MONILIA VAGINITIS

I. **Definition:** An infection of the vagina caused by the fungus *Candida albicans.*

II. **Etiology**

   A. Monilia is a normal inhabitant of the digestive tract. It is usually kept in check in the vagina by the inhospitable acidic environment, caused by lactic acid produced by lactobacilli in the epithelial cells. This keeps the pH of childbearing women between 4.0 to 4.5 and prepubertal girls and postmenopausal women at approximately 5.0.

   B. Monilia thrives in high glucose environment. Therefore, any situation that renders the vagina higher in glucose and/or increases the pH to 4.5 to 5.0 will encourage growth of monilia. Situations that seem to predispose to monilia include:

   1. Those related to high glucose:
      a. Pregnancy
      b. Use of oral contraceptives containing progestin
      c. Diabetes mellitus
      d. High-glucose diet
      e. Obesity
   2. Those that increase vaginal pH:
      a. Too frequent douching
      b. Too frequent use of oils, jellies, creams, which upset the vaginal pH
      c. Possibly a high-stress lifestyle
      d. Use of broad-spectrum antibiotics (including Flagyl), which destroy the lactobacilli that make the vagina acidic

   C. Monilia can grow on skin and mucous membranes including:
   1. Vulva and vagina
   2. Penis and scrotum
   3. Mucous membranes of oral cavity. This is called thrush and can be transmitted to the newborn while passing through the birth canal of an infected mother.

III. **Clinical Features**

   A. Signs and symptoms
   1. Intense burning and itching of vulva and vagina
   2. Red patchy excoriated appearance of vulva
   3. Discharge that resembles cottage cheese, thick white or yellow.
   4. Curdy patches that stick to vaginal mucosa and cervix
   5. Dyspareunia, dysuria, urinary frequency
   6. May have typical "yeasty" odor
   7. Symptoms often develop premenstrually

   B. Microscopic findings on wet mount
   1. Filaments with budding spores

2. Pseudo hyphae; may be more apparent on potassium hydroxide (KOH) slide
    C. Can be identified on Pap smear
IV. **Management**
    A. Treatment of active infection
        1. Terazol vaginal cream or suppositories for 3 to 7 days
        2. Monistat vaginal cream or tablets, one full applicator or tablet at bedtime for 7 days or two tablets at bedtime for 3 days
        3. Gyne-Lotrimin cream or tablets, one full applicator or tablet at bedtime for 7 days or two tablets at bedtime for 3 days
        4. One Diflucan 150 mg orally; it takes 2 to 5 days to obtain complete relief
        5. To relieve itching and burning
            a. Sitz baths in cool or tepid water three times a day
            b. Dry vulva with a blow dryer on lower setting after sitz bath.
            c. Apply extra vaginal cream or ointment to affected areas.
    C. Educate regarding prevention measures.
        1. Avoid douching, oils, creams, and perfumed products, such as scented or deodorized tampons or pads and deodorized soaps.
        2. Use white toilet paper, rather than colored.
        3. Avoid refined sugar in the diet.
        4. Avoid excessively stressful life-style, get plenty of sleep and rest.
        5. Wear panties with a cotton crotch. Avoid the use of nylon panties, pantyhose, and tight slacks. Do not wear underwear to bed.
        6. A beginning monilia infection can be avoided by inserting acidophilus tablets, plain yogurt, or boric acid capsules into the vagina to restore the normal acidic pH. Soak a tampon in the yogurt and insert it in the vagina. Try one of these methods nightly for a few nights. If the infection worsens, medication is needed.
        7. If put on a course of broad-spectrum antibiotics, may try preventive methods used in number 6.
    D. If patient has frequent or chronic infections:
        1. Examine the male partner. He may be harboring the fungus and infecting the woman, especially if uncircumcised. Apply antifungal cream to penis and under foreskin for 7 days.
        2. Consider screening for diabetes, HPV of the cervix.
    E. Treatment of frequent or recurrent infections:
        1. Order Diflucan 150 mg to be taken orally 3 to 5 days before period every month for 3 to 6 months.
        2. Nizoral 200 mg orally, every day for month. May repeat for 2 months, do SGOT before continuing past 3 months.
    F. A pregnant patient with a history of frequent infections should be assessed for active infection near term by history and wet prep. It is desirable to treat even a subclinical infection at term to avoid transmission of thrush to the neonate at the time of delivery.

MULTIPLE PREGNANCY

I. **Definition:** A pregnancy involving two or more fetuses.
II. **Incidence**
   A. Approximately 2% of births in the United States are multiple.
   B. Most involve twins; triplets occur in 1 of 7600 pregnancies.
   C. Multiple births higher than triplets are rare, but the incidence is rising due to the increasing use of gonadotropins to treat women with ovulatory failure and new methods of returning fertilized eggs (zygotes) to the uterus.
III. **Etiology:** Racial or family tendency to twinning increases the likelihood of dizygotic pregnancy, but not in monozygotic pregnancy.
IV. **Clinical Features**
   A. History
      1. History of recent infertility problem treated with fertility drugs
      2. Familial history of twins
   B. Signs and symptoms
      1. Large-for-dates uterine size, fundal height, and abdominal girth associated with rapid uterine growth during the second trimester. Especially significant if early uterine size was consistent with dates.
      2. Inexplicable excessive weight gain
      3. Abdominal palpation reveals three or more large parts and/or multiple small parts, especially in the third trimester when these are more readily felt.
      4. Auscultation of more than one FHT
   C. Potential complications
      1. Polyhydramnios is more common.
      2. The incidence of pre-eclampsia is increased fivefold.
      3. Anemia is prevalent.
      4. Postpartum hemorrhage (PPH) is more common due to overdistention of the uterus
      5. Prematurity is greatest cause of fetal morbidity and mortality in multiple gestations
      6. Fetal mortality is quadrupled in twin pregnancy. Risk to the second twin is twice that of the first.
      7. Congenital malformations are more common.
      8. Malpresentation, premature rupture of membranes (PROM), and cord prolapse are more common.
      9. Dystocia in labor and caesarean section are more likely.
   D. Discomforts
      1. Discomforts associated with large intrauterine volume
         a. Dyspnea
         b. Heartburn
         c. Abdominal pain and/or itching

2. Excessive weight gain due to:
   a. Increased volume of uterine contents
   b. Increased water retention
   c. Polyhydramnios
   d. Overeating
3. Complaints of fetal overactivity are frequent.
4. Increased fatigue and hunger

V. **Management**
   A. At initial visit, ask about personal or family history of twins.
   B. If at any time signs and symptoms develop, confirm or rule out with sonogram.
   C. If diagnosed, consult; collaborative management is possible for twins.
   D. Usual antepartum management
      1. Increase oral iron to 120 mg elemental iron per day.
      2. Increase folic acid to 1 mg per day.
      3. Offer referral to dietitian. Increase protein intake to 120 gm/day and add 500 extra calories to diet.
      4. Office visits every 2 weeks after 24 weeks
      5. Weekly NST after 32 weeks
      6. Consider vaginal exam at every office visit after 24 weeks to check for cervical changes that would indicate impending premature labor.
      7. Advise patient to stop work outside the home by 24 weeks and to restrict travel.
      8. Advise frequent rest periods after 30 weeks.
      9. Provide support, reassurance, and teaching regarding associated discomforts and potential dangers.
      10. Monthly sonogram for growth and positions.
   E. Management during labor and delivery
      1. Collaborative management
         a. Management is the physician's prerogative
         b. Certified nurse-midwife may deliver first baby if vertex.
         c. Certified nurse-midwife may assist with second infant as necessary.
      2. Obtain ultrasound on admission to hospital for fetal position.
      3. IV or heparin lock is mandatory in labor.
      4. Fetal monitoring of both babies is mandatory in labor.

NON-STRESS TEST

I. **Definition**
   A. A test of fetal condition in which fetal movements are recorded and concomitant fetal heart rate changes are monitored.

II. **Indications:** All patients at risk for placental insufficiency
   A. Hypertension: At 32 weeks, at least weekly as long as hypertension is a concern, then biweekly at 36 weeks
   B. Gestational diabetes: Weekly after 32 weeks
   C. Possible IUFGR biweekly after diagnosis
   D. Postdates: Biweekly after 40 weeks
   E. Marked decrease in fetal movements: at once, then as indicated depending on results
   F. Previous stillbirth: Weekly after 32 to 34 weeks, if undelivered, biweekly after 40 weeks.
   G. Any other combination of factors suggesting an increased risk of placental insufficiency, such as total weight gain below 15 pounds at 36 weeks EGA, heavy smoker, drug abuse, etc.

III. **Management**
   A. Reactive test
     1. Baseline heart rate between 120 and 160 beats per minute
     2. Four or more fetal movements within a 20 minute tracing
     3. Heart rate acceleration of at least 15 beats per minute with a duration of 15 seconds or more above the baseline rate two times in 20 minutes
   B. Nonreactive test
     1. Physician should be consulted for any non-stress test that does not meet the criteria designated above.
     2. Depending on the situation, the patient could be sent out to eat and return later for another test or she may be sent to the hospital to:
        a. Try another NST
        b. Do a nipple stimulation test
        c. Do a contraction stress test (CST)

PAPANICOLAOU (PAP) SMEAR

I. **Definition:** A cervical cytologic exam introduced in 1941, instrumental in reducing the incidence and mortality rates for cervical cancer. The Bethesda system for classification of the results of Pap smears in the one that is most used. However, because some locations still use the older systems, a comparative overview is given in Table 3-4.

II. **Etiology**
   A. Cervicitis caused by STDs, yeast, bacteria
   B. Reparative changes from trauma to the cervix
   C. Vaginal atrophy in menopause
   D. HPV
      1. Found in 97% to 98% of cervical cancers
      2. Contributing factors that increase the chance of exposure to HPV are:
         a. Unprotected sex
         b. Early age at first intercourse
         c. Multiple sex partners
         d. High-risk male partner
         e. Exposure to other STDs

Table 3-4. Overview of Classification Systems for Pap Smears*

Original "Class" System	Modifications (1960s, 1970s)	Bethesda System (1988, 1991)
Class I—normal	Normal	Normal
Class II—slightly suspicious for malignancy	Atypical cells but below the level of cervical neoplasia	Atypical squamous cells of undetermined significance
Class III—moderately suspicous for malignancy	Dysplastic cells present consistent with intraepithelial neoplasia; often graded as cervical intraepithelial neoplasia (CIN) I–III	Low-grade squamous intraepithelial lesion; equivalent to changes associated with human papilloma virus and CIN I
Class IV—highly suspicious for malignancy	Carcinoma in situ (CIN III)	High-grade squamous intraepithelial lesion; equivalent to CIN II–III
Class V—diagnostic for malignancy	Invasive cancer	Invasive cancer

*These systems are not directly interchangeable.
From Lemcke DP, Pattison, J, Marshall LA, Cowley DS. *Primary Care of Women.* Norwalk, CT: Appleton & Lange, 1995;72. Reprinted with permission.

E. Contributing factors that lower the immune system
　1. Pregnancy
　2. Debilitating diseases
　3. Cigarette smoking
　4. Malnutrition

III. **Management**
　A. Normal—repeat in 1 year
　B. ASCUS or class II
　　1. May be atypical because of inflammation. Treat offending organism if identified by Pap or try to identify organism. If unable to identify a specific organism, treat with a vaginal cream, such as Cleocin vaginal cream or Triple Sulfa vaginal cream, for general infections. Readminister Pap in 2 to 3 months.
　　2. Class II with mild dysplasia—do colposcopy.
　　3. Class II with atypica consistent with HPV, koilocytosis, or parakytosis must have a colposcopy.
　C. Certical intraepithelial neoplasia (CIN) I or class III
　　1. Colposcopy as soon as possible
　　2. If colposcopy, therapy will be based on colposcopy and biopsy findings. Therapy may include observation or laser in pregnancy. If not pregnant, LEEP, cone biopsy, cryosurgery, or laser
　D. CIN II to III or class IV: Refer to physician management.

NOTES

PEDICULOSIS PUBIS (CRABS)

I. **Definition and Etiology:** An infestation of the vulva caused by crab louse, *Phthirus pubis,* or its nits. It is contracted via contact with an infested person or object, such as clothing, bed linens, upholstered furniture.

II. **Clinical Features**
   A. Patient may have no symptoms or may notice lice or nits on body hair.
   B. Diagnosis is made by finding the lice or nits attached to body hair
      1. Usual location is pubic hair
      2. Occasionally the following body hair may be involved:
         a. Thighs, trunk
         b. Eyelashes, eyebrows
         c. Axilla
         d. Scalp

III. **Management**
   A. If pregnant or breastfeeding
      1. Stop-X, RID, or other OTC medications may be used. Contraindicated in patients with ragweed sensitivities
         a. Apply sufficient liquid to completely wet hair and skin of any infected areas. Avoid contact with eyes and mucous membranes.
         b. Leave on for 10 minutes.
         c. Wash and rinse with plenty of warm water.
         d. Use a clean fine-tooth comb to remove nits and dead lice.
         e. If head hair is treated, follow with shampoo.
         f. If retreatment is necessary, do not exceed two applications within 24 hours.
      2. If first trimester, limit to one treatment if possible. Treat as many times as necessary in second and third trimesters.
   B. In not pregnant or breastfeeding, use Kwell 1% cream or lotion (4 ounces).
      1. Bathe or shower before beginning treatment and dry with a clean towel.
      2. Apply lotion or cream over entire body from neck down.
      3. Leave on for 24 hours.
      4. Wear clean clothes and sleep in clean bed linen during the 24-hour treatment.
      5. Reapply to hands after each washing during 24-hour treatment.
      6. Take a cleansing bath 24 hours after application, **no sooner.**
      7. If scalp is involved:
         a. Use Kwell shampoo.
         b. Leave on for 5 minutes before rinsing.
         c. Shampoo with regular shampoo.

- d. Use a clean fine-tooth comb to remove nits and dead lice.
  8. Pubic, underarm, and other infested body hair should be combed to remove nits and dead lice.
C. Other considerations
  1. Crabs can live over a month on inanimate objects.
    a. All combs, hairbrushes, curler, etc. should be cleaned with Kwell.
    b. All clothing and bed linens should be washed in hot water with detergent and dried in an electric dryer. A commercial washer is better because the water is hotter.
    c. Clothing and bed linen that cannot be washed should be dry cleaned.
    d. Upholstered furniture, beds, and pillows should be cleaned.
  2. If eyelashes are involved, apply occlusive ophthalmic ointment before treatment.
  3. Retreatment may be necessary in 1 week because eggs hatch that were not killed during treatment.
  4. Sexual partner(s) within preceding month also need treatment.

NOTES

PLACENTA PREVIA

I. **Definition:** A placenta that is implanted in the lower pole of the uterus. This implantation can be:
   A. Total or complete: The entire cervical os is covered by the placenta.
   B. Partial: Only a portion of the os is covered.
   C. Marginal: Edge of placenta is at the edge of os.
   D. Low-lying: Edge of placenta is almost at edge of os.

II. **Incidence:** One in 200 births.

III. **Etiology**
   A. Factors that affect the localization of implantation:
      1. Early or late fertilization
      2. Variability in the implantation potential of the blastocyst
      3. The receptivity and adequacy of the endometrium
   B. In multiple pregnancies because the placental surface is increased in size
   C. Tendency to avoid implantation on uterine scar, for example, previous caesarean section
   D. Rate increases proportional to increase in parity. The endometrium is changed at previous placental site; the blastocyst tries to attach where no placenta has been before.
   E. Rate increases in older women.
   F. Rate increases in diabetes, possibly because the placenta is larger than usual.

IV. **Clinical Features**
   A. Signs and symptoms
      1. Painless vaginal bleeding
      2. Sudden onset of bleeding without warning
      3. Occurs during third trimester
      4. Malpresentation or malpositions because the fetus must accommodate itself to the presence of the placenta
   B. Complications
      1. Hemorrhage and resulting shock
      2. Prematurity of the fetus
      3. Postpartum hemorrhage due to bleeding at the site of placental implantation where the uterine muscle fibers contract less effectively.
      4. Sheehan's syndrome and clotting defects may occur but are more common in placental abruption.

V. **Management**
   A. Do not do vaginal exams! A placental vessel may be ruptured and result in massive hemorrhage.
   B. Diagnosis can be made by ultrasound.

C. If diagnosis is made early in pregnancy, placenta may migrate up in the uterus as the uterus enlarges.
    1. Follow-up with serial ultrasounds until the placenta is well away from the cervical os. If the placenta still encroaches on the os at 32 weeks, refer to a physician.
    2. Instruct the patient to call at the first sign of any vaginal bleeding.
D. Consult with physician immediately upon diagnosis of total, partial, or marginal placenta previa after 20 weeks of pregnancy.
E. See that any unsensitized Rh(D)-negative patient receives a RhoGAM injection after each bleeding episode to prevent sensitization from possible mixing of D positive fetal blood with maternal blood. The usual dose is 1 vial, which is adequate for a transfusion of up to 15 ml fetal blood into the maternal circulation. The dosage should be larger if it is possible that more than 15 ml was transfused. A Kleinhauer-Betke test can be done to determine the amount of fetal blood in the maternal circulation.
F. A woman with diagnosed total or partial placenta previa is kept on limited activity or bedrest and observed closely until the baby is mature or until a serious bleeding episode occurs that necessitates immediate delivery. Delivery is by caesarean section since the placenta is blocking the cervical os and prevents vaginal descent of the fetus.

VI. **Patient Education**
A. Explain the causes, location of the placenta, and possible problems.
B. The patient is to call at the first sign of bleeding. She should inform the hospital or person she talks to of the previa diagnosis.
C. Patients with a total or partial previa should remain at home on limited activity.
D. No intercourse
E. Information should be given on caesarean section in case this is or becomes necessary.

NOTES

PNEUMONIA

I. **Definition:** Inflammation of the lung parenchyma in which the affected part is consolidated.
II. **Etiology**
   A. Often follows common viral upper respiratory illness.
   B. Two thirds of cases are bacterial.
   C. Other common causes are mycoplasma pneumonia, varicella, and streptococcus.
III. **Clinical Features**
   A. Fetal considerations: If any of the below are protracted enough or severe enough, the fetus is adversely affected; mortality can be up to 30%.
      1. Hypoxia secondary to maternal hypoxia—the fetus tolerates it better than the mother due to:
         a. High glycogen content of fetal tissues
         b. Ability of the fetus to use anaerobic metabolic pathways
      2. Hypoglycemia—there is a decrease in blood glucose in the mother, partly due to hyperthermia and partly due to the disease process.
      3. Hyperthermia
   B. Maternal considerations—by type of pneumonia
      1. Influenza pneumonia
         a. Signs, symptoms, and course of disease
            (1) First 6 to 12 hours—prodromal phase
               (a) Malaise
               (b) Myalgia
               (c) Headache
               (d) Pain on ocular movement
               (e) Chilling, fever
               (f) Nasal congestion
               (g) Mild sore throat
            (2) Second or third day—clinical deterioration
               (a) Cough with purulent sputum if bacteria are present
               (b) Diffuse bilateral crepitant basilar inspiratory rales
               (c) Occasionally, pleuritic chest pain
               (d) Dyspnea
               (e) Hemoptysis
            (3) Fourth day
               (a) Cyanosis secondary to pulmonary decompensation
               (b) Shock secondary to cardiovascular collapse
               (c) Fetal death, then maternal death
         b. Diagnosis: Presumptive, based on clinical course and radiograph

2. Varicella-zoster pneumonia
   a. Signs, symptoms, and course of disease
      (1) Respiratory symptoms develop 2 to 5 days after cutaneous lesions appear. Initial and sometimes only manifestation is a dry nonproductive cough.
      (2) In more severe disease:
         (a) Cough becomes productive after 36 to 48 hours; mucoid sputum, which may be blood-streaked, or frank hemoptysis may occur.
         (b) Bilateral acinonodular infiltrates on radiograph
         (c) Dyspnea, tachypnea, cyanosis, chest pain
   b. Diagnosis
      (1) Other signs of varicella-zoster (chickenpox or shingles) in woman or family
      (2) Definitive: Serological confirmation or virus isolation
      (3) Chest radiograph
3. Streptococcus pneumonia
   a. Signs, symptoms, and course of disease
      (1) Initial onset is dramatically sudden.
         (a) Productive cough—sputum watery at first, then rapidly becomes purulent grayish-green, then characteristic rust color
         (b) Fever
         (c) Malaise
      (2) Extension of disease
         (a) Pleuritic chest pain
         (b) Chills with tremor
         (c) Shortness of breath, orthopnea, tachypnea, cyanosis
         (d) Fine crepitant rales
         (e) Tachycardia
   b. Diagnosis
      (1) Presence of encapsulated lancet-shaped diplococci on gram stain smear of sputum
      (2) Radiograph: Significant expansion of involved pulmonary parenchyma

IV. **Management**
   A. See Guidelines on page 99 for management of specific signs and symptoms.
      1. Colds and flu
      2. Nasal congestion
      3. Coughs
      4. Sore throat
      5. Headache

B. The patient should be seen in the office or emergency room if th lowing signs and symptoms are present. Elicit onset, duration, cou se, and any self-treatment measures for each:
   1. Fever greater than 102°F
   2. Pain on ocular movement
   3. Severe chest pain
   4. Severe dyspnea, orthopnea, or tachypnea
   5. Purulent or bloody sputum
   6. Severe sore throat that interferes with swallowing or breathing
   7. Any of the conditions in section A above that do not respond to conventional therapy
C. Physical exam
   1. Inspect throat for infection, edema, abscess
   2. Palpate submental, submaxillary, tonsillar, and cervical lymph nodes.
   3. Observe for dyspnea, tachypnea, orthopnea, tachycardia, cyanosis.
   4. Take temperature.
   5. Percuss and auscultate lungs for wheezes, rales, rhonchi, decreased breath sounds, and areas of consolidation.
D. Labwork
   1. Throat culture if throat infected
   2. Sputum culture as necessary
   3. CBC if fever
E. Penicillin therapy is the treatment of choice.

NOTES

POLYHYDRAMNIOS

I. **Definition:** An excessive amount of amniotic fluid.
II. **Etiology**
   A. Multiple gestations, especially with monozygotic twins
   B. Diabetes
   C. Erythroblastosis
   D. Fetal malformations
      1. Gastrointestinal tract, for example, esophageal atresia or some other abnormality that would prohibit fetal swallowing of amniotic fluid
      2. Central nervous system anomalies, for example, anencephaly, meningomyelocele
III. **Clinical Features**
   A. Complications
      1. Fetal malpresentation
      2. Placental abruption
      3. Problems in labor
         a. Premature labor
         b. Premature rupture during labor
         c. Uterine dysfunction during labor
         d. Cord prolapse
         e. Postpartum hemorrhage secondary to atony from uterine overdistention
      4. Baby small for gestational age
   B. Signs and symptoms
      1. Uterine enlargement, abdominal girth, and fundal height far beyond that expected for gestational age.
      2. Tenseness of the uterine wall, making it difficult or impossible to:
         a. Auscultate fetal heart tones.
         b. Palpate the fetal outline and parts.
      3. Auscultation of a uterine fluid thrill
      4. If severe, mechanical problems such as:
         a. Severe dyspnea
         b. Lower extremity and vulvar edema
         c. Pressure pain in back, abdomen, and/or thighs
         d. Nausea and vomiting
IV. **Management**
   A. Ultrasound for definitive diagnosis
   B. If diagnosis confirmed by ultrasound, consult with physician. Collaborative management is possible. Usual management:
      1. Advise patient of associated conditions and complications.

2. Order repeat scan to observe for fetal abnormalities
3. Do daily fetal activity counts (FAC) and weekly non-stress test (NST).
4. Advise restriction of activities (bedrest if severe).
5. Plan delivery at hospital with level III nursery if labor starts before 35 weeks.
6. Instruct patient to call at first sign of labor.
7. If moderate to severe: Consult, consider induction of labor with prostaglandins gel or pitocin.
8. Notify physician if patient is hospitalized for labor.
9. Avoid artificial rupture of membranes (AROM) in labor unless vertex -1, -2 and well applied to the cervix.
10. IV or heparin lock is mandatory in labor because of increased likelihood of postpartum hemorrhage.
11. Fetal monitor is mandatory in labor.
12. Notify pediatrician or neonatal nurse practitioner when delivery is imminent.

NOTES

POSTMATURITY

I. **Definition:** Any pregnancy that goes to the end of the 42nd week. Some sources are currently defining postmaturity as any pregnancy that goes to the end of the 41st week.

II. **Incidence**
   A. If not induced, 12% of all pregnancies would reach the 43rd week.
   B. If not induced, 4% of all pregnancies would reach the 44th week.

III. **Etiology**
   A. Malfunction in the labor-starting mechanism
   B. A variation in the time it takes for fetus to mature
   C. More common with anacephaly

IV. **Clinical Features:** Problems associated with postmaturity
   A. Fetal dysmaturity syndrome
      1. Cause: Placental insufficiency
      2. Signs and symptoms
         a. Low weight in relation to length
         b. Little subcutaneous fat, baggy skin
         c. Vernix scant or absent
         d. Hair and nails long
         e. Skin dry and peeling, especially on hands and feet
         f. Skin, nails, and cord gold- or green-colored from meconium staining
         g. Reduced amount of amniotic fluid, thick with meconium
   B. Dystocia—risk of shoulder dystocia in labor because of fetal macrosomia
   C. Increased perinatal mortality from:
      1. Anoxia secondary to placental insufficiency
      2. Difficult birth due to dystocia
      3. Higher incidence of meconium aspiration

IV. **Management**
   A. Establish clear EDC as early in pregnancy as possible.
      1. Ultrasound before 12 weeks, especially of the crown-rump length, tends to be more accurate for dating purposes and should be given more weight in decision making.
   B. Discuss labor stimulation and post-dates management at 40 to 41 weeks. Labor stimulation includes:
      1. Increase walking and other activity
      2. Sexual excitement—intercourse/orgasm
   C. Advise patient to keep fetal movement log beginning at 39 weeks.
   D. At 40 to 41 weeks:
      1. Begin biweekly NSTs per guidelines.

Table 3-5. Bishop's Score

	Bishop's Score			
	0	1	2	3
Dilatation (cm)	0	1–2	3–4	5–6
Effacement (%)	0–30	40–50	60–70	80+
Station	−3	−2	−1	+1 +2
Consistency	Firm	Medium	Soft	
Position	Posterior	Mid	Anterior	

A score of four or greater is considered positive and yields a successful induction rate of 80% to 90%. A score of nine is almost failproof.

      2. Evaluate cervix for ripeness according to Bishop score (Table 3-5). If ripe:
         a. Consider stripping the membranes.
         b. If Bishop score greater than 9, consider induction.
         c. Consider prostaglandin gel if cervix is unripe.
      3. If patient desires to go into labor naturally and is greater than 41 weeks EGA, consider biophysical profile.
  E. Consult with physician for any of the following:
      1. Abnormal NST or oxytocin challenge test (OCT)
      2. Ultrasound showing oligohydramnios
      3. Biophysical profile less than 8
      4. Induction

POSTPARTUM HEMORRHAGE

THIRD STAGE HEMORRHAGE

I. **Definition:** Blood loss of 500 ml or more between the time the baby is delivered and the time the placenta is delivered.
II. **Etiology:** Partial separation of the placenta
III. **Management**
   A. Prevent by managing third stage properly.
      1. Do not massage the uterus during third stage.
      2. Do not pull the placenta. Allow physiologic separation, which may take up to 30 minutes.
   B. If third stage hemorrhage occurs:
      1. Thoroughly massage the uterus to contract and complete placental separation, while applying mild cord traction to effect delivery (Brandt-Andrews maneuver)
      2. Instruct assistant to start IV or insure patency if already in place. (Ringer's lactate is best.)
      3. If there is difficulty delivering the placenta and/or hemorrhage continues, have assistant call for physician immediately.
      4. If physician has not yet arrived and hemorrhage continues, perform manual removal of the placenta. If time and conditions permit, have epidural redosed or give patient 2 mg Stadol or Demerol 50 mg IV before manual removal is attempted.
      5. If the placenta is out but bleeding continues, perform bimanual compression.
         a. Order 10 to 20 units Pitocin to current IV if not already given
         b. If not improving, see Fourth Stage Hemorrhage Management Guidelines on page 201.
      6. If signs and symptoms of shock develop:
         a. Infuse Ringer's lactate solution (RL) rapidly.
         b. Place patient flat with legs slightly elevated.
         c. Give oxygen per mask.
         d. Keep patient warm, cover with warm blankets.
         e. Continue monitoring vital signs.

FOURTH STAGE HEMORRHAGE

I. **Definition:** Blood loss of 500 ml (some references use 650 ml) or more between the time the placenta is delivered and 24 hours after.
II. **Etiology**
   A. Uterine atony due to:
      1. Primary atony
      2. Overdistended uterus
         a. Multiple gestation

b. Large baby
   c. Polyhydramnios
  3. Exhaustion of uterine muscle
     a. Multiparity
     b. Prolonged labor
     c. Use of oxytocin in labor
  4. Inability of the uterus to contract properly:
     a. Precipitous labor, delivery, or both
     b. Uterine myomas
     c. Full bladder
 B. Trauma and lacerations
  1. Episiotomy. Blood loss can reach 200 cc normally. When arterioles or large veins are cut or torn, the amount of blood loss can be considerably more.
  2. Lacerations of the vulva, vagina, or cervix
  3. Ruptured uterus, possibly from a previous caesarean scar.
  4. Uterine inversion
  5. Puerperal hematomas
 C. Retained placental fragments or clots

III. **Management**
 A. Preventive techniques
  1. Clamp bleeding vessels immediately to conserve blood.
  2. Avoid a prolonged interval between performance of episiotomy and delivery of the baby.
  3. Avoid undue delay from birth of the baby to repair of episiotomy or lacerations.
  4. Routinely inspect upper vaginal vault and cervix.
  5. Start repair above apex to avoid failure to secure a bleeding vessel there.
  6. Routinely inspect placenta for missing parts and broken vessels. Be aware of trailing membranes at time of delivery of the placenta.
  7. If there is reason to believe placental fragments are retained, medicate as necessary, manually explore uterus, inform physician as necessary.
 B. Consult with physician if:
  1. Physician was not notified during the emergency
  2. Bleeding persists or returns
  3. Symptoms of hypovolemia, such as dizziness, faintness, tachycardia, are unrelieved with hydration.
  4. There is a significant drop in the hematocrit (<27%).
 C. If there is a significant drop in hematocrit, start patient on iron supplements and educate regarding dietary sources of iron and folic acid.
 D. Prophylactic antibodies should be given if the uterus was explored.
 E. Be alert for signs of postpartum infection.

F. Blood or blood products should never be given except as a last resort and after consulting.

LATE POSTPARTUM HEMORRHAGE

I. **Definition:** Blood loss of 500 ml or more after the first 24 hours of delivery and within 6 weeks.

II. **Etiology**
   A. Retained fragments of placenta; infection usually follows.
   B. Subinvolution of the uterus and placental site
   C. Uterine myoma, especially when submucosal
   D. Hematoma or reproductive tract laceration
   E. Idiopathic, tendency to recurrence
   F. Late detachment of thrombi at the placental site with reopening of the vascular sinuses
   G. Abnormalities in the separation of the decidua vera
   H. Intrauterine infection, leading to dissolution of the thrombosis in the vessels

IV. **Management**
   A. Usual treatment
      1. Oxytocics
         a. Methergine 0.2 mg orally every 4 hours for 6 doses
         b. May need to be admitted to hospital for D&C if presently hemorrhaging.
      2. Antibiotics if infection exists
   B. Immediate management
      1. Support the lower uterine segment and express clots.
      2. Check the consistency of the uterus.
         a. If atonic, massage it.
         b. If no response, do bimanual compression.
         c. Give oxytocics and/or ergots listed here in order of preference:
            (1) Pitocin 10 to 20 units to 1000 cc IV fluids
            (2) Methergine 0.2 mg intramuscularly if no history of hypertension
            (3) Prostin suppositories per vagina, uterus, or rectum.
            (4) If still bleeding administer Hemabate 1 amp IM every 5 minutes three times. Give first dose 10 minutes post prostin.
         d. Send someone to call physician.
         e. Continue bimanual compression.
         f. Have assistant monitor vital signs and watch for signs of shock.
      3. If bleeding is not under control, have assistant get type and cross if not already done.

4. If uterus is well-contracted and bleeding continues, look for lacerations.
   a. If first or second degree lacerations of vagina or perineum, repair.
   b. If lacerations of cervix or third or fourth degree lacerations of vagina or perineum:
      (1) Clamp any bleeders and wait for physician.
      (2) If physician still has not arrived and hemostasis is not attained, repair as necessary to attain hemostasis.
5. If signs of shock develop:
   a. Infuse LR rapidly.
   b. Place patient flat with legs slightly elevated.
   c. Give oxygen per mask.
   d. Keep patient warm, cover with blankets.
   e. Have assistant monitor vital signs.
6. In extreme cases, consider the following:
   a. Injection of oxytocin directly into the uterus with Iowa trumpet
   b. Aortic compression
   c. Alert OR in case a D&C or hysterectomy are necessary

C. Follow-up management
   1. Obtain hematocrit:
      a. Twelve hours after delivery
      b. Twenty-four hours after delivery

NOTES

PREMATURE RUPTURE OF MEMBRANES

I. **Definition:** Rupture of membranes before the onset of labor.
II. **Etiology**
   A. Preterm labor
   B. Chorioamnionitis twice as frequent in PROM
   C. Malposition or malpresentation of fetus
   D. Factors due to cervical damage
      1. Prior cervical instrumentation (eg, therapeutic abortion (TAB), LEEP, etc.)
      2. Increasing parity with possible damage to the cervix during previous deliveries
      3. Incompetent cervix
   E. Previous history of PROM twice or more
   F. Factors due to maternal weight
      1. Overweight before pregnancy
      2. Low weight gain during pregnancy
   G. Cigarette smoking during pregnancy
   H. Advanced maternal age possibly because the membranes are less strong than in young mothers
   I. Recent coitus
III. **Management**
   A. Prevention
      1. Treat gonococcus, chlamydia, bacterial vaginosis.
      2. Discuss smoking in pregnancy and support efforts to cut down or quit.
      3. Encourage adequate weight gain in pregnancy.
      4. May discuss abstaining from coitus in the last trimester if any of the predisposing factors are present.
   B. Anticipatory guidance: Inform the following patients prenatally that they should call immediately if membranes rupture.
      1. Conditions in which ruptured membranes could result in cord prolapse
         a. Presenting part other than vertex
         b. Polyhydramnios
      2. Active herpes
      3. Previous history of beta hemolytic streptococcus
   C. If membranes have ruptured:
      1. Instruct patient to go to hospital or office.
      2. Document rupture.
         a. Obtain careful history. Attempt to establish a time of rupture
         b. If gross rupture:

(1) While patient is lying supine, apply fundal pressure to see if it elicits a gush of fluid from the vagina.

(2) Wet a cotton swab with fluid and smear on a slide to assess ferning under a microscope.

(3) Apply some fluid to Nitrazene paper. If positive, consider diagnostic if patient has not had recent sex, is not bleeding, and has not been examined vaginally using K-Y Jelly.

 c. If uncertain of rupture and/or signs of possible infection, perform sterile speculum exam.

(1) Attempt to assess Bishop score of cervix (see Table 3-5).

(2) Do culture of cervix only if signs of infection.

(3) Obtain another specimen of fluid with a sterile swab to smear on slide to assess ferning under microscope.

 d. If gestation is less than 37 weeks or patient has a herpes II outbreak, refer to physician.

D. Conservative management
  1. Most labor starts within 24 to 72 hours of rupture.
  2. Possibility of infection is less if nothing is put into the vagina but sterile speculum; **no vaginal exams.**
  3. Waiting involves close monitoring of patient.
     a. Temperature four times a day—if it rises significantly and/or reaches 100.4°F two antibiotics are necessary and delivery needs to be accomplished.
     b. Observe vaginal discharge: foul odor, purulent or yellowish appearance indicates infection.
     c. Note uterine tenderness and irritability and report any changes.

E. Aggressive management
  1. Prostaglandin gel may be used after consulting with physician
  2. May require serial Pitocin induction if cervix is unfavorable
  3. Some wait 12 hours for labor. If none, Pitocin is started.
  4. Involves need for IV, fetal monitor
  5. Increased risk of caesarean if induction ineffective
  6. If decision depends on inducibility of cervix, assess Bishop score (see Table 3-5) after speculum exam. If decision is then made to wait for labor, **no more** exams are to be done, either digital or speculum, until labor starts or an induction is started.
  7. Obtain CBC if rupture documented. Repeat every other day until delivery or more often if signs of infection.
  8. Obtain NST following rupture; be alert for fetal tachycardia, which is one of the first signs of infection.
  9. Begin induction after consult with physician if:
     a. Significant rise in maternal temperature
     b. Fetal tachycardia develops
     c. Foul lochia
     d. Significant uterine irritability or tenderness

- e. Vaginal culture shows beta hemolytic streptococcus
- f. CBC indicates elevated white count (shift to left).
- **F.** Management of labor more than 24 hours after rupture
  1. Spontaneous labor
     - a. Obtain patient's temperature every 2 hours, initiate antibiotics if fever develops.
     - b. Internal monitoring suggested
     - c. Notify obstetrician and pediatrician or neonatal nurse practitioner.
     - d. Cultures per guidelines
  2. Induction of labor
     - a. Per routine orders after consult with physician
     - b. Obtain patient's temperature every 2 hours.
     - c. Antibiotics: Guidelines differ. Many give 1 to 2 g of ampicillin IV or 1 to 2 g of Mefoxin IV every 6 hours prophylactically. Others monitor maternal temperature and FHT rate and use that information to determine when antibiotics may be needed.

NOTES

PREMATURITY

I. **Definition:** Labor that occurs after the 20th week and before the 37th week of gestation
II. **Incidence:** 7% of all pregnancies
III. **Etiology**
   A. In 66% of cases, the cause is never determined.
   B. Maternal factors
      1. Debilitating medical disorders
         a. Cardiovascular disease
         b. Renal disease
         c. Severe hypertension
         d. Poorly controlled diabetes
         e. Any other serious disease
      2. Abdominal surgery involving uterine displacement and/or manipulation when pregnant
      3. Maternal injury
      4. Pre-eclampsia or eclampsia
      5. Uterine anomalies
      6. Pelvic sepsis or tumors
      7. Infections
         a. Viral
            (1) Cytomegalovirus
            (2) Herpes simplex
            (3) Hepatitis
         b. Pyelonephritis
         c. Chorioamnionitis caused by infection
      8. Cervical incompetence
      9. Two or more previous abortions
   C. Placental factors—abruption
   D. Fetal factors
      1. Multiple gestation
      2. Polyhydramnios
      3. Large baby
      4. PROM
      5. Infection (rubella, toxoplasmosis, etc.)
IV. **Management**
   A. If previous history of premature labor:
      1. Explore possible causative factors.
      2. Consider obtaining screening cultures especially if:
         a. History of more than one previous premature labor

b. History of any of the associated infections
   c. History of previous unexplained stillbirth
  3. Cervical exams in office each antepartal visit
B. If patient presents in labor:
  1. Determine if labor is true or false.
     a. If contractions are irregular, infrequent, or painless, probably Braxton-Hicks. Instruct patient to:
        (1) Increase fluid intake.
        (2) Lie down.
        (3) Call back if contractions increase in regularity, frequency, or pain.
     b. If contractions are regular, frequent, or uncomfortable, instruct patient to come into office or to labor and delivery for external monitoring.
  2. Fetal fibronectin (fFN) may be assessed by sterile speculum exam and cervico-vaginal swab.
     a. Normally present in cervico-vaginal fluid after 20 weeks EGA.
     b. It is released as a result of compromise in the fetoplacental membrane structure or strength.
     c. Eighty-seven percent of those with a positive test will deliver within 7 days.
     d. Ninety-nine and one half percent of those with a negative fFN will deliver over 7 days after the test; 97% will deliver over 14 days after a negative test.
  3. If patient is in true labor, consult with physician. Usual treatment:
     a. Labor will usually not be stopped if any of the following conditions are present.
        (1) Before 20 or after 35 weeks' gestation
        (2) Three to four centimeters dilation and 50% to 75% effaced
        (3) Maternal complications, such as hypertension or diabetes
        (4) Fetal complication, such as IUFGR
        (5) Placental complications, such as abruption
        (6) Premature rupture of membranes: May want to stop labor for 24 hours to mature fetal lungs
        (7) Chorioamnionitis
     b. If chance of delivery is high and patient is less than 35 weeks, she should be transferred to a hospital with level III nursery due to need of neonatal intensive care for infant.
     c. If labor is to be stopped, follow standard hospital guidelines for terbutaline or magnesium sulfate as ordered by the comanaging physician.
     d. Factors to be considered if delivery is inevitable.
        (1) If there is a chance that at least 24 hours might elapse before delivery, and patient is less than 33 weeks' gestation, consider Betamethasone therapy to increase surfactin production and mature the fetal lungs.

- **(2)** Keep analgesia to a minimum. Narcotic depression is exaggerated in the premature baby.
- **(3)** Electronic fetal monitoring is indicated
- **(4)** Cut a large episiotomy; avoid trauma to the fetal head.
- **(5)** The pediatrician or neonatal nurse practitioner should be called to be present for the delivery.

NOTES

PRURITUS IN PREGNANCY

I. **Definition:** Generalized body itching during pregnancy with or without accompanying jaundice
II. **Etiology**
   A. Not definite but could possibly be caused by:
      1. Obstetric cholestasis
      2. High estrogen levels
      3. Elevated serum bile salts
   B. More common in multiple gestations
   C. Subsides soon after delivery
III. **Clinical Features**
   A. Generalized or local body itching especially the abdomen and feet
   B. Mild jaundice
   C. Elevated serum bilirubin levels
   D. Rash usually beginning on the trunk and abdomen and spreading to include the entire body
   E. Usually begins after 28 weeks of pregnancy
IV. **Differential Diagnosis**
   A. Hepatitis
      1. Previous history of hepatitis, jaundice
      2. Family member with hepatitis
      3. Working/living in a high exposure area
      4. IV drug use
   B. Liver disease
      1. Rare with no previous history or history of hepatitis
      2. Get SMAC-20 plus CBC to test liver function if any doubt.
   C. Scabies
      1. Look for rash or papules in skin folds.
      2. Ask if other family members have same symptoms.
   D. Allergic reactions, poison ivy topical medication, etc.
      1. Look for accompanying hives and/or rash
      2. History of recent exposure to allergen
      3. Itching is in area exposed, which is not usually the abdomen or feet
   E. Skin disease
      1. Previous history
      2. Lesions not characteristic of simple excoriation from scratching
   F. Cholestasis of pregnancy
      1. Recurs in each pregnancy (familial)
      2. High level of alkaline phosphate and serum bile acids

3. Pruritus, jaundice may be present. No anorexia or malaise
4. Last trimester

V. Management

A. When a patient presents with pruritus, make differential diagnosis
B. Consult if any doubt about diagnosis.
C. Simple pruritus gravidarum is managed symptomatically.
   1. Avoid scratching; it may lead to secondary infection due to excoriation of the skin.
   2. Try antipruritic lotion, such as Calamine or Benadryl.
   3. Try anesthetic ointment or spray. such as Americaine.
   4. Apply ice packs to affected area.
   5. In severe cases, may try Benadryl 25 to 50 mg orally every 4 to 6 hrs as necessary; use sparingly.
   6. Mild excoriation may respond to hydrocortisone 1% cream.
D. In severe skin excoriation, probable allergic response or skin disease, refer to dermatologist.
E. See Skin Conditions in Pregnancy on page 226 and Rashes on page 228 for further information.

NOTES

PUERPERAL INFECTION

I. **Definition:** Any infection of the genital tract during the puerperium, accompanied by a temperature of 100.4°F or higher on any 2 of the first 10 days postpartum exclusive of the first 24 hours.

II. **Clinical Features**
   A. Predisposing factors
      1. Length of labor
      2. Duration of ROM
      3. Retained products of conception
      4. Abdominal delivery
      5. Number of vaginal exams during labor
      6. Anemia
   B. Symptoms
      1. Fever
      2. Malaise
      3. Abdominal pain
      4. Uterine tenderness
      5. Purulent or foul-smelling lochia
   C. Differential diagnosis
      1. Dehydration
         a. Occurs in the first 24 hours after delivery.
         b. Should not last more than 24 hours.
         c. Temperature should not go over 100°F.
      2. Breast engorgement
         a. Occurs on the third to fifth day postpartum; when milk is coming in, breasts feel warm, full, uncomfortable.
         b. Should not last more than 12 hours.
         c. Temperature should not go over 100.4°F

III. **Management**
   A. Physical exam
      1. Check temperature and pulse.
      2. Possible upper respiratory infection or pneumonia
         a. Inspect throat for infection, swelling, drainage.
         b. Palpate lymph nodes of the head and neck for adenopathy.
         c. Auscultate lungs for rales, rhonchi, wheezes.
      3. Possible mastitis: Observe breast for localized redness, tenderness.
      4. Possible wound infection: observe perineal or abdominal wound for redness, tenderness, warmth, swelling, purulent drainage, abscess formation.
      5. Possible endometritis
         a. Palpate uterus for tenderness.

b. If other findings suggestive of endometritis, do speculum and bimanual exam, get endocervical cultures, and assess lochia for odor and characteristics.
   6. Possible UTI or pyelonephritis
      a. Check for costovertebral angle tenderness (CVAT).
      b. Question regarding signs and symptoms of UTI.
      c. Obtain clean catch or catheterized urine.
   7. Possible thrombophlebitis
      a. Presence of Homans's sign
      b. Observe calves for any reddened areas that are warm to touch, and swelling
B. Labwork—do as indicated by history and physical.
   1. Usual standard workup for most common causes
      a. Urinalysis and culture and sensitivity. Postpartum UTI is often asymptomatic, so this is fairly routine.
      b. Endometrial cultures
      c. Blood cultures
      d. CBC with sedimentation rate and differential
   2. Other labwork that may be done if history and physical indicate:
      a. Culture of perineal or abdominal wound
      b. Culture of breast milk
      c. Culture of sputum, throat, or both
C. Treatment
   1. Avoid use of antipyretics unless fever is over 101°F.
   2. If fever under 101°F in first 24 hours, force fluids at 200 cc/hr (orally or IV) and retake temperature in 2 to 3 hours. If still elevated, do workup.
   3. If fever under 100°F at time milk is coming in, encourage frequent breastfeeding and warm compresses to breasts. Monitor temperature every 2 to 3 hours. If fever gets higher and/or persists longer than 12 hours, do work-up.
   4. If tests are normal, treat as indicated. Otherwise, consult physician.

RASHES

I. **Acne**
   A. Clinical picture
      1. Skin comedones, papules, pustules
      2. Severe cases include cysts, abscesses, pits, and scars
   B. Rule out:
      1. Pyoderma
      2. Drug eruptions
   C. Treatment
      1. Wash with medicated soap three times per day.
      2. Drying lotions or gels with benzoyl peroxide 5% to 10%, Persa-Gel 5%, Desquam-X 5% to 10%, every day or twice a day
      3. Antiseborrheic shampoo if indicated
      4. Tetracycline 500 mg orally four times a day for 7 to 10 days, then 500 mg every day or twice a day if protected against pregnancy
      5. Retin-A—not recommended while pregnant
      6. Dermatology—consult if severe or not responsive to above.
   D. Patient education
      1. Well-balanced diet
      2. Use no oil, grease, or creamy cosmetics on skin.
      3. No hair lotions or creams
      4. Expect exacerbations during periods of stress and menses.
      6. Keep hands off face.

II. **Athlete's Foot (Tinea Pedis)**
   A. Clinical picture
      1. Itching, scaling feet
      2. Acute form—vesicles on soles, side of feet, and between toes
      3. Chronic form—lesions are dry and scaly.
      4. Toenails may be thickened with debris under nail.
   B. Rule out:
      1. Contact dermatitis
      2. Psoriasis
      3. Bacterial infection
   C. Treatment
      1. Blisters should be snipped and drained, and edges of blisters should be trimmed to avoid fungi from spreading under edges.
      2. Apply Desenex foot powder or Tinactin cream or lotion to affected area twice a day until 1 week after lesion heals.
   D. Patient education
      1. Air dry feet 20 minutes three times a day.

2. Dry between toes after bathing.
3. Wear well-ventilated shoes or sandals with exposure of feet to the air when possible.
4. Wear rubber sandals in community showers or bathing places.

III. Contact Dermatitis
A. Clinical picture
1. Patient complains of pruritus and burning.
2. Erythematous papules and vesicles
3. Linear streaks of erythema or vesicles are seen where offending item has been in contact with skin areas.

B. Types
1. Contact dermatitis from allergic reaction
2. Contact dermatitis due to poison oak or poison ivy

C. Treatment
1. Avoid item(s) that caused problem.
2. Prescribe Atarax, Benadryl, or Zyrtec for pruritus.
3. If there is weeping, perform a cold compress soak for 20 minutes and apply Calamine lotion after each soak.
4. If there is no weeping, apply 1% hydrocortisone cream three times a day until lesions resolve.

D. Patient education
1. Remove offending item(s).
2. Trim fingernails and keep them clean and short.
3. If from poison oak or poison ivy, wash all clothing, shoes, etc. that have come in contact with the plant.
4. Wear loose-fitting clothing.
5. Consult with or refer to physician if there is involvement of eyes.

IV. Eczema
A. Patient presents with:
1. Pruritus
2. Family history of allergic diseases or atopic dermatitis
3. History of asthma and allergic rhinitis

B. Clinical picture
1. Infancy
   a. Lesions—erythematous and papular to scaling or vesicular, which may progress to oozing and crusting
   b. Located usually on cheeks, scalp, postauricular area, neck, and extensor surface of forearms and legs
2. Childhood
   a. Lesions—more dry, papular, scaling eruptions with hypopigmentation
   b. Located on flexor surfaces of wrists and on antecubital and popliteal areas

3. Adolescence and adulthood
   a. Lesions—dry, thickened skin, with accentuation of normal lines and folds, often with hyperpigmentation
   b. Located usually on flexor areas of extremities, eyelids, back of neck, and dorsum of hands and feet
C. Rule out:
   1. Seborrheic dermatitis
   2. Fungal infections of the skin
   3. Contact dermatitis
   4. Irritant dermatitis
D. Treatment
   1. Antihistamine for pruritus
      a. Benadryl 25 to 50 mg orally every 6 hours or Benadryl lotion/ointment
      b. Atarax 25 to 100 mg three to four times a day
      c. Vistaril 50 to 100 mg IM
   2. Severe, weeping lesions; refer to dermatologist.
   3. After acute exudative phase has been controlled, apply hydrocortisone cream 1%, 0.5% four times a day.
   4. Apply Eucerin cream, Aqua-Aquaphor, or Lubriderm lotion after bath or shower to seal in moisture.
   5. Antibiotics (topical or systemic) for secondary bacterial infection
E. Patient education
   1. Avoid hot water.
   2. Short showers are best or one to two baths per week and for no longer than 5 minutes.
   3. Avoid soaps and bubble baths. Use a mild soap like Dove or Neutrogena for cleaning dirty areas.
   4. Avoid wool, and starched or rough clothing.
   5. Keep fingernails short.
   6. Pat skin dry and avoid rubbing skin with washcloth.

V. **Folliculitis**
   A. Clinical picture
      1. Patient complains of mild to severe pain at site.
      2. Lesions are pinhead-sized or slightly larger pustules surrounded by a narrow area of erythema. Many pustules are located in same area.
      3. Location of lesions are usually seen on scalp, axilla, or extremities.
      4. *Staphylococcus aureus* most often is the causative organism.
   B. Rule out:
      1. Tinea of scalp
      2. Contact dermatitis
   C. Treatment

1. Warm compresses of tap water four times a day
2. Topical application of Neosporin ointment. If more than three lesions, consider orally antibiotics.
3. Folliculitis of scalp—Selsun Suspension twice per week
4. Consult doctor for cases involving fever and cellulitis.

D. Patient education
1. Wash affected area with soap and water. Apply hot compresses for 20 minutes four times a day.
2. Avoid use of hair oils, bath oils, or suntan oils.
3. Return in 1 week if lesions do not clear or before if fever is present.

VI. Furuncles and Carbuncles

A. Clinical picture
1. Patient complains of mild to severe pain at site.
2. Inflammatory reaction with pain and tenderness
3. Lesions may be 2 cm or more.
4. May be single or multiple, chronic and recurrent
5. Often resolve by necrosis and spontaneous drainage

B. Rule out:
1. Impetigo
2. Foreign objects with associated infection
3. Insect bites
4. Diabetes, immune deficiency if there is a recurrence of furuncles or carbuncles

C. Treatment
1. Hot moist compresses for 20 minutes four times a day
2. Topical antibiotic ointment, such as Neosporin
3. Incision and drainage when the necrotic white area appears at top of nodule
4. Systemic antibiotics for severe furunculosis
5. Surgical consult if lesion is extensive. May need incision and drainage plus packing with iodoform or sterile gauze.

D. Patient education
1. General hygiene
2. If other family members affected, have them evaluated.

VII. Hives (Urticaria)

A. Obtain history.
1. New foods
2. Medication
3. Family history of allergies
4. Recent illness
5. Previous occurrence

B. Clinical picture

1. Patient complains of itching.
2. Red or raised plaques of welts with sharp borders, which may vary in size and number, and are usually located on trunk and extremities.
3. Lungs are clear and patient is not wheezing.

C. Rule out:
1. Erythema multiforme
2. Multiple insect bites—fleas, mosquitoes
3. Contact dermatitis

D. Treatment
1. If immediate and severe, check heart rate and BP, and give Epinephrine 1:1000, 0.3 to 0.5 ml subcutaneous (SQ) for adults. **Consult physician immediately.** May follow with Benadryl 25 to 50 mg orally every 4 to 6 hours.
2. Mild or moderate—Benadryl 25 to 50 mg orally every 4 to 6 hours or Zyrtec 10 mg orally every day. A divided dose of 5 mg orally of Zyrtec may provide better 24-hour coverage.
3. Soaks in tub of cool water or oatmeal bath will provide additional antipruritic effect.

E. Patient education
1. Instruction on danger signs: call if difficulty breathing.
2. Inform if allergic reaction to medication; rash may worsen over the next 1 to 2 days and take several weeks to resolve.
3. Observe for recurrence and note commonalities so source can be identified.

VIII. Impetigo

A. Clinical picture
1. Patient complains of pruritus.
2. Vesicular eruptions, containing serous fluid that becomes purulent and surrounded by areas of erythema
3. Pustules rupture, dry centrally, and form a honey-colored crust.
4. Lesions vary in size from a few millimeters to several centimeters.

B. Rule out:
1. Noninfected insect bites
2. Herpes simplex
3. Chickenpox
4. Other vesicular or ulcerating skin lesions

C. Treatment
1. Culture lesion if necessary for diagnosis.
2. Crusts are soaked with warm water compresses 5 to 10 minutes before removing them at least three times a day.
   a. Warm soaks with Betadine or Dial soap may be used.
   b. Apply Neosporin ointment to lesions after removing crusts.

3. Systemic antibiotic can be given if patient has more than a couple of lesions.
    a. Penicillin is the treatment of choice for 10 days.
    b. Erythromycin if allergic to penicillin for 10 days.
D. Patient education
    1. No one else should use patient's washcloth, towel, or bed linen.
    2. Trim fingernails
    3. Other family members having skin lesions need evaluation.

IX. **Molluscum Contagiosum**
   A. Clinical picture
      1. Characterized by skin-colored, smooth, waxy, umbilicated papules, 2 to 10 mm in diameter.
      2. Transmitted by direct contact
   B. Rule out:
      1. Acne
      2. Infected hair folliculus/sebaceous glands
   C. Treatment
      1. Remove the core of the papule with a needle.
      2. Wash with a medicated soap.
      3. Take Neosporin or other antibiotic ointment twice a day and as necessary.

X. **Moniliasis**
   A. Patient may have:
      1. Pruritus at site
      2. Monilia vaginitis
      3. History of diabetes
      4. History of birth control pill use
      5. Breastfeeding infant may have thrush.
   B. Clinical picture
      1. Well-defined, red, eroded patches with scaly, pustular, or pustulovesicular diffuse borders, commonly occurring in the intertriginous areas, such as the axillae, on or around the breasts, between fingers and toes.
      2. White patches on oral mucosa, which usually bleed when removed.
   C. Rule out:
      1. Seborrheic dermatitis
      2. Other fungal skin infections
   D. Treatment
      1. Apply antifungal cream such as Monistat or Lotrimin twice a day for 2 weeks.
      2. Oral: Use Nystatin Oral Suspension, 100,000 units/ml 2 ml, four times a day for 1 to 2 weeks. Place 1 ml on each side of mouth so medication is in contact with lesion for as long as possible. If pre-

ferred, may give Nizoral 100 mg, 1 orally every day. Continue treatment for 2 weeks after lesions are gone.
  E. Patient education
     1. Instructions for proper cleaning and drying of affected areas
     2. Instruct on method of transmission.
XI. **Seborrheic Dermatitis**
  A. Clinical picture
     1. Pruritus
     2. Skin flaking
     3. Redness and scaly skin eruptions, which may be dry or greasy
     4. Location of lesions often start at the scalp (cradle cap in infants) and progress to eyebrows, eyelids, nasolabial folds, postauricular folds and external auditory canal, presternal area, and diaper area.
     5. May be associated with acne
  B. Rule out:
     1. Tinea capitis or corporis
     2. Psoriasis
     3. Contact dermatitis
     4. Candidiasis
  C. Treatment
     1. Mild cases—nonprescription dandruff shampoo
        a. Head and Shoulders shampoo
        b. Selsun Blue shampoo
     2. Moderate cases—Selsun Suspension twice a week for 2 weeks, then once a week. Leave on scalp 15 to 30 minutes before washing off.
     3. Refer to dermatologist.
  D. Patient education
     1. Instructions for brushing hair and removing crusts
     2. No Vaseline, grease, or oil on scalp
     3. It is not contagious and will not cause baldness, there are seasonal variations.
     4. Chronic—will get better and worse
     5. Is familial

ROUND LIGAMENT PAIN

I. **Etiology**
   A. The round ligaments attach on either side of the uterus just below and in front of the insertion of the fallopian tubes, cross the broad ligament in a fold of peritoneum, pass through the inguinal canal, and insert in the anterior (upper) portion of the labia majora on either side of the perineum. They are supporting structures for the uterus.
   B. As the uterus grows in pregnancy, the ligaments become stretched and often contract, resulting in sharp pain along the side of the abdomen, just above the groin area, usually accentuated by sudden movements, coughing, lifting, etc.

II. **Differential Diagnosis**
   A. PID
   B. Appendicitis
   C. Kidney stone
   D. Gallbladder or other GI disease
   E. UTI
   F. Placental abruption
   G. Labor

III. **Management**
   A. Explain reason for pain and reassure patient.
   B. Comfort measures
      1. Avoid sudden movement, turn slowly to side and push up rather than trying to sit straight up from lying down.
      2. Apply local heat.
      3. Try a change of activity.
      4. Maternity girdle may be helpful.
      5. Support uterus with a pillow when sitting or lying down.
      6. May take Tylenol g every 4 hours as necessary for pain
   C. If no relief with above measures, obtain pelvic ultrasound.
   D. Instruct patient to call if sharp abdominal pain does not subside within 30 minutes; it may be something besides round ligament pain.
   E. If all tests are negative and discomfort continues, refer to physician, physical therapist, or chiropractor as needed.

RUBELLA

I. **Definition and Etiology:** An acute exanthematous disease caused by the rubella virus and marked by enlargement of lymph nodes. It is of importance because of the high incidence of fetal abnormalities. It is also called German measles or 3-day measles.

II. **Clinical Features**
   A. Course of the disease
      1. Spread by aerosol dissemination from nasopharynx and/or oropharynx. Virus is shed for at least 10 to 14 days after rash appears.
      2. Course of Infection

         Incubation period—time frame: 11 to 14 days after exposure
         Postauricular adenopathy—time frame: 7 days before rash appears until 1 to 2 weeks
         Maculopapillary rash begins on upper thorax of face and spreads downward—time frame: 11 to 17 days after exposure, lasts 3 days
         Virus shedding—time frame: 10 to 14 days after rash appears
         Antibody formation—time frame: first appears with rash, peaks 24 to 28 days later, declines twofold to eightfold after a few weeks

      3. Arthralgia and sometimes arthritis are not uncommon complications if strain is particular virulent.
   B. Rubella virus is well adapted to humans, causes little morbidity or mortality except to fetus.

III. **Management**
   A. All prenatal patients need a rubella screen on the initial visit unless there is documentation that one was done during the present pregnancy.
   B. If antibody positive (>1:10), no treatment is needed. If titer greater than 1:1000, repeat as soon as possible to rule out lab error.
      1. If still elevated, repeat in 3 weeks to rule out potential convalescent serum.
      2. If repeat serum is decreased, a recent rubella infection is indicated. Consult with physician.
   C. If antibody negative (<1:10), discuss getting immunization postpartum.
      1. Should get informed consent for immunization
         a. Woman must not be pregnant at time of vaccination and should not become pregnant for at least 3 months after vaccination.
         b. About 10% of those vaccinated develop transient arthritis. Risks to others in her environment is minimal.
      2. If sterilization is performed immediately postpartum, vaccination is not necessary.

D. If possible exposure or infection occur during pregnancy:
  1. Obtain titer.
     a. If titer drawn on or before rash, repeat 7 to 10 days later. If eightfold increase, infection occurred.
     b. If titer drawn within 5 days of onset of rash, repeat 7 to 10 days after onset of rash and compare the two titers. If the second is significantly increased over the first, be suspicious of rubella even though the increase will not be as much as eightfold.
     c. If titer drawn more than 5 days after onset of rash is high in conjunction with postauricular adenopathy, or much higher than original initial titer, be suspicious of rubella.
     d. If uncertain of exposure or physical signs, repeat titer in 3 weeks. If there is a significant increase, be suspicious of rubella.
E. If any suspicion of rubella exposure in a patient who was negative at the initial screening, inform patient of potential risks to fetus. There is an inverse relationship between the age of the fetus at the time of maternal infection and the severity of anomalies.
  1. Effect on fetus according to age
     a. If fetus is of 3-to-7-weeks gestation at time of exposure, death usually results due to serious anomalies.
     b. If fetus is of 8-to-13-weeks gestation at time of exposure, deafness is the principal defect.
     c. Teratogenic manifestations are limited to organ systems with a limited capacity to regenerate in the first trimester.
        (1) Cataracts are characteristic.
        (2) Congenital heart disease
        (3) Hearing problems
        (4) Growth retardation
        (5) Clotting disorders
        (6) Mental retardation
        (7) Chromosomal abnormalities
     d. Serious manifestations after 13 weeks fetal age at time of exposure are rare, but growth retardation can occur even though organogenesis is complete. The expanded congenital rubella syndrome includes:
        (1) Hepatosplenomegaly
        (2) Pneumonitis
        (3) Hepatitis
        (4) Encephalitis
        (5) Lesions of the long bones
        (6) Anemia
        (7) Thrombocytopenic purpura
  2. The fetus does not produce antibodies because the mother's antibody response suppresses that of the fetus. So babies will shed virus at birth and 50% will shed until 6 months of age.

SCABIES

I. **Definition and Etiology:** A skin eruption caused by a mite, *Sarcoptes scabies*. Contracted via contact with an infested person or object, such as clothing, bed linen, upholstered furniture.

II. **Clinical Features:** Patient presents with an intensely pruritic papular or excoriated erythematous skin rash involving:
   A. The webs of the fingers and toes
   B. Anterior wrist surface and the backs of the knees
   C. Axillae
   D. Trunk, especially at the waistline
   E. Genitalia and buttocks, especially gluteal and inguinal folds

III. **Management**
   A. Diagnosis
      1. Confirmed by microscopic findings
         a. Scrape lesions.
         b. Transfer the scraping to a slide.
         c. Apply a drop of oil and a coverslip.
         d. Look for the mite and/or its eggs or fecal pellets.
      2. Microscopic evidence is frequently difficult to find. Therefore, diagnosis is often made on the basis of:
         a. History, especially of other family members with similar signs and symptoms
         b. Characteristic appearance and distribution of skin lesions
         c. Ruling out other dermatologic conditions
   B. Treatment
      1. If patient is pregnant or breastfeeding, use Eurax cream, 6 ounce tube.
         a. Massage into skin of body from chin down, especially folds and creases.
         b. Reapply 24 hours later. Do not bathe first.
         c. Take a cleansing bath 48 hours after the last application.
         d. Consider a second application after 4 to 5 days for particularly heavy infestations.
      2. If patient is not pregnant or breastfeeding, may also use Eurax cream or may use Kwell 1% lotion or cream.
      3. Treatment consideration:
         a. During treatment, thoroughly launder all clothing and bed linen with detergent and hot water and dry in an electric dryer. Dry clean clothes that cannot be washed. Clean all upholstered furniture.
         b. Consider treating other family members, especially if symptomatic.
         c. Sexual partner(s) should be evaluated and treated.

d. Advise patient that itching may continue for several weeks after adequate treatment.
      1. Antipruritic lotion, such as Caladryl
      2. Anesthetic ointment or spray, such as Americaine
      3. Applying ice packs to the affected area
      4. In severe cases, may try Benadryl 25 to 50 mg orally as necessary. Use sparingly.

NOTES

SKIN CONDITIONS IN PREGNANCY

I. **Physiologic**
   A. Definition: Physiologic alterations in the skin common in pregnancy
   B. Etiology: Hormonal changes during pregnancy—fetoplacental production, stimulation or changes in metabolism may increase the availability of estrogens, progesterone, androgens, and other hormones in the mother's body.
   C. Clinical Features
      1. Hyperpigmentation
         a. Incidence: 90%
         b. Stimulated by estrogen, progesterone, melatonin-stimulating hormone
         c. Darkening of linea nigra, genitalia areolae, nipples, freckles, nevi, recent scars
         d. Regresses after delivery
      2. Chloasma, mask of pregnancy
         a. Seen frequently in pregnant women
         b. Seen in 5% of nonpregnant women on BCPs
         c. Consists of blotchy, irregular hyperpigmentation on cheeks, forehead, upper lip, and neck. Exacerbated by sun and wind.
         d. Regresses after delivery. Type caused by BCPs may persist
      3. Hirsutism/alopecia
         a. During pregnancy, hair growth is stimulated.
         b. Postpartum hair re-enters resting phase.
         c. Many hairs shed within 3 to 6 months causing thinning hair and a dandruff looking scalp.
         d. Patient education consists of reassurance, shampoo for dandruff.
      4. Striae
         a. Appear in 90% of patients
         b. Probably caused by increased adrenocortical activity
         c. No clear correlation with abdominal girth
         d. Appear as pink or purple atrophic bands, which fade to white
         e. Pruritis at site is a frequent complaint. Antipruritic ointment and lotions help.
      5. Vascular distention, proliferation, and instability
         a. Congestion of the vestibule and vagina
         b. Palmar erythema
         c. Varicosities, involve saphenous, vulval, hemorrhoidal veins
         d. Arterial spiders (65% of Caucasians, 11% of African American)
         e. Pallor, facial flushing, hot and cold sensations, are secondary to vasomotor instability.

- f. Hyperemia and hypertrophy of gums
- g. Most vascular changes regress postpartum.

II. **Skin Disorders Unique to Pregnancy**
   A. See Table 3-6.

III. **Skin Manifestations of Diseases That Affect Pregnancy**
   A. Coxsackie B Enterovirus
      1. Rash is typically maculopapular exanthem that resembles rubella.
      2. Diagnosis
         a. Viral culture of throat and rectum
         b. Acute and convalescent IgM, IgG
      3. Fetal problems
         a. Main concern is maternal infection in third trimester, resulting in neonatal exposure. The risk to the neonate is less if the interval to delivery is 4 to 6 weeks. This allows the mother to develop immunity, which is passively transmitted to her fetus.
         b. Rare cases of congenital cardiac defects have been reported.
   B. Fifth disease—"Slapped face" syndrome
      1. Caused by parvovirus B-19
      2. Epidemic late winter and spring
      3. Spread by nasal droplets
      4. Incubation 4 to 14 days
      5. Signs and symptoms are general malaise, fever, URI. Infection wanes as rash appears. Rash starts on the face and resembles slapped cheeks. It then spreads to the trunk and extremities.
      6. Diagnosis
         a. B-19 parvovirus antibody. IgM can be detected 3 days after symptoms. Starts to fall in 30 to 60 days, may persist at low levels 4 to 6 months.
         b. Parvovirus B-19 IgG can be detected after 7 days of illness, persists for year.
         c. Since labs report both IgM and IgG, need only draw blood once between 4 days and 4 weeks of the onset of symptoms.
      7. Management of positive infection during pregnancy
         a. Serial hemoglobin and hematocrit to detect aplastic anemia resulting from bone marrow suppression
         b. Serial ultrasound to watch for fetal hydrops. The virus destroys fetal erythroid precursors. Fetal death, usually 1 to 12 weeks after infection, is caused by severe anemia, congestive heart failure. Babies treated in utero for severe anemia often do well with no lasting problems.
   C. Varicella (chickenpox, varicella-zoster)
      1. Clinical features
         a. Varicella-zoster virus causes both chickenpox and herpes zoster. *(text continues on page 230)*

Table 3-6. Skin Disorders Unique to Pregnancy

Disorder	Frequency	Clinical Characteristics	Histopathology	Perinatal Outcome	Treatment	Comments
Pruritus gravidarum	Common (1%–2%)	Onset third trimester intense pruritus; generalized; excoriations common	Noncharacteristic; excoriations common	Perinatal morbidity increased	Antipruritics, cholestyramine	Possibly a mild form of cholestatic jaundice; recurs in subsequent pregnancy. Common in nulliparas; seldom recurs in subsequent pregnancy.
Pruritic urticarial papules and plaques of pregnancy	Common (0.25%–1%)	Onset second or third trimester; intense pruritus; patchy or generalized, abdomen, thighs, arms, buttocks; erythematous papules, urticarial papules and plaques	Lymphocytic perivascular infiltrate; negative immunofluorescence	No adverse effects	Antipruritics, emollients, topical steroids, oral steroids if severe	Common in nulliparas; seldom recurs in subsequent pregnancy
Papular eruptions (prurigo gestations and papular dermatitis)	(1:300–1:2400)	Onset second or third trimester; localized or generalized; 1–5 mm pruritic papules; excoriations common	Lymphocytic perivascular infiltrate; parakeratosis, acanthosis; negative immunofluorescence	Possibly unaffected	Antipruritics, topical steroids, oral steroids if severe	Prurigo gestations localized to forearms and trunk; papular dermatitis generalized; does not recur in subsequent pregnancy

Herpes gestations	Rare (1:50,000)	Onset second or third trimester, sometimes 1–2 wk postpartum; severe pruritus; abdomen, extremities, or generalized; urticarial papules and plaques, erythema vesicles, and bullae	Edema; infiltrate of lymphocytes, histiocytes, and eosinophils; C_3 and IgG deposition at basement membrane	Possibly increased preterm birth; transient neonatal lesions (5%–10%)	aaaaaa	Also associated with gestational trophoblastic disease; exacerbations and remissions during pregnancy common; postpartum exacerbations very common; recurrence in subsequent pregnancies more severe
Impetigo herpetiformis	Rare	Onset third trimester; local then generalized; erythema with marginal sterile pustules; mucous membranes involved; systemic symptoms	Micro abscesses	Maternal sepsis common	Antibiotics, oral steroids	Possibly pustular psoriasis; persists for weeks to months postpartum; may recur with subsequent pregnancy

From Cunningham FG, McDonald P, Grant N, Levent K, Gilstrap L. *Williams Obstetrics*. 19th ed. Norwalk, CT: Appleton & Lange, 1993; 1261. Reprinted with permission.

b. Chickenpox: Incubation period for primary infection is 10 to 20 days. Lesions begin on trunk and spread. Lesions progress from macules to vesicles and crust over. New lesions appear for 3 to 5 days, causing severe itching.
   c. Herpes zoster recurrent form. Lesions develop along nerves.
2. Fetal effects
   a. Maternal illness: 5 to 21 days before delivery results in mild chickenpox in newborn.
   b. Maternal illness 4 days before to 48 hours after delivery may result in severe disseminated disease in baby, 30% fatal.
   c. Maternal infection earlier in pregnancy may cause fetal skin scarring, muscle atrophy, hypoplastic extremities, club feet, cortical atrophy, encephalitis.
3. Maternal effects—watch for maternal pneumonia.
4. Labwork
   a. Isolation of virus from lesion first 4 days
   b. Fluorescent antibody membrane antigen (FAMA) or enzyme-linked immunosorbent assay (ELISA) to determine immune status
   c. Antibody found 2 weeks following illness. Increase in titer over previous value indicates recent infection. Antibody disappears over time.
   d. Check to see if IgG present.
5. Prevention
   a. Avoid exposure to persons with known active disease if immunity uncertain.
   b. If negative history of disease or not immune can give immunity within 96 hours of exposure. Give VLIG, varicella/zoster immune globulin IM. One vial of 125 units/10 kg of weight (maximum = 625 units).

NOTES

SORE THROAT

I. **Clinical features**
   A. History
      1. Onset, duration, course, and self-treatment measures
      2. Previous history of frequent sore throat or strep throat
      3. Associated symptoms
         a. Cough
         b. Nasal congestion
         c. Fever, myalgia
         d. Nausea/vomiting, diarrhea
         e. Headache
         f. Lung involvement
      4. Is it severe enough to interfere with eating or drinking?
   B. Physical exam
      1. Inspect throat for infection, swelling, abscess
      2. Palpate submental, submaxillary, tonsillar, and cervical lymph nodes. If swollen and tender, indicative of infection.
      3. Percuss and auscultate lungs for decreased breath sounds, wheezes, rales, rhonchi, areas of consolidation. If present, indicative of lung involvement.
      4. If temperature elevated, indicative of infection
   C. Labwork
      1. If throat infected, obtain culture.
      2. If febrile, consider CBC.

II. **Management**
   A. Soothe throat.
      1. Saline or mouthwash gargles
      2. Chloraseptic spray
      3. Cough lozenges, especially those with local anesthetic
   B. If throat culture indicates bacterial infection, treat with appropriate antibiotic. Do not prescribe antibiotic without obtaining results of a throat culture.
   C. If sore throat is interfering with adequate nutrition, hydration, or both:
      1. Counsel regarding need for at least 8 cups of liquid per day.
      2. Advise soft, cool, easily swallowed foods that supply nutritional needs, such as jello, custard, or ice cream. Take a nutritional supplement such as Ensure.

SYPHILIS

I. **Definition:** An acute and chronic infectious venereal disease.
II. **Etiology**
   A. Syphilis is caused by *Treponema palladum*, a spirochete that infects mucous membrane.
   B. Length of incubation period from time of exposure to appearance of primary chancre depends on the number of organisms established at the time of infection and how long it takes them to replicate. Spirochetes take 33 hours to replicate as compared with minutes for bacteria.
      1. Incubation for the primary stage is 10 to 90 days after contact, averaging 21 days. Signs and symptoms resolve spontaneously in 3 weeks without treatment.
      2. Incubation for the secondary stage is 17 days to 6 months after contact, averaging 2.5 months. If not treated, signs and symptoms resolve spontaneously in 2 to 8 weeks, with an average of 4 weeks.
      3. Latent stage begins after the secondary lesions are gone.
   C. A person is contagious when lesions, either primary or secondary, are present.
   D. Early antibody response is IgM. Within 2 weeks it changes to IgG.
III. **Clinical Features**
   A. Acquired syphilis
      1. Primary phase:
         a. Primary lesion is a chancre: A small papule that forms at the portal of entry and breaks down to form a superficial painless ulcer that lasts about 5 weeks and heals spontaneously. Lesions can be so mild as to escape detection. May be single or multiple.
         b. Dissemination from the portal of infection to the lymph nodes occurs in about 70%, causing satellite buboes, enlarged tender firm lymph nodes.
      2. Secondary phase results from hematogenous dissemination from drainage of regional lymph nodes drainage. Characterized by:
         a. A generalized bilateral nonpruritic painless skin rash anywhere on the body, but especially on mucous membranes, palms of hands, and soles of feet. Rash may be either or all:
            (1) Flat, coppery-colored maculas
            (2) Erythematous scaly papules
            (3) Pustules
         b. Involvement in the mouth appears as white erosions called "mucous patches."
         c. Intertriginous confluent condyloma latum in moist areas of the body, such as the vulva and perianal region. Look like a group of small, flat warts covered with a grayish exudate; are highly infectious. Do not confuse with condylomata acuminata, the external warts caused by HPV.

d. Systemic symptoms are common.
   (1) Generalized lymph adenopathy
   (2) Fever, malaise, lethargy, headache
   (3) Anorexia, weight loss
   (4) Alopecia anywhere on the body
3. Latent phase takes place after the manifestations of secondary syphilis disappear without treatment. The spirochete lies dormant in the body and manifests itself several years later as multi-organ degeneration. Diagnosed by lab tests in the absence of clinical manifestations, especially with a history of known exposure or history of primary or secondary lesions.

B. Congenital syphilis
  1. Is primarily a reflection of inadequate prenatal care
  2. Placenta appears pale gray, large in relation to baby's weight, and often is fibrotic.
  3. Fetal and neonatal effects
     a. Increase in spontaneous abortion, stillbirth, neonatal death
     b. Effects in relation to treatment:
        (1) If not treated, heart defects and "snuffles" are main defects.
        (2) If mother treated before 16 weeks, infection of baby is probably prevented because the spirochete does not usually cross the placental barrier before that time.
        (3) If mother treated after 16 weeks, course of syphilis is arrested in baby but defects that already exist will remain.
        (4) If mother has latent syphilis, the baby can be infected but infectivity decreases with the duration of the mother's infection. If the mother has had latent syphilis over 4 years, the baby will probably not be affected.

IV. **Lab Tests**
  A. Rapid plasma reagin (RPR)
    1. Not a titer; does not give antibody level
    2. Once positive, remains positive for life
    3. Is more sensitive than VDRL in picking up active infection during early stages
  B. VDRL
    1. Once positive, remains positive for life
    2. Can be rendered positive by any number of febrile diseases, as well as syphilis
    3. False positive about 1:8
    4. Is a titer, unlike the RPR
    5. Low level indicates effective treatment, a high level indicates active infection.
    6. Once a patient has had syphilis, all the blood tests will be positive. The VDRL is most useful for follow-up or rediagnosis.
  C. Fluorescent treponema antibody (FTA)

1. Specific to syphilis because it identifies the treponema organism
2. Once positive, remains positive for a long time, possibly for life.
   D. Dark field microscopic exam of serum from a lesion identifies the treponema organisms.

V. **Management**
   A. All patients should have an RPR or VDRL ordered at initial prenatal visit.
      1. If RPR positive, the patient may or may not have syphilis.
         a. Order FTA, if no previous history of syphilis.
            (1) If FTA negative, assume patient does not have syphilis if no clinical signs or symptoms are present.
            (2) If FTA positive, obtain VDRL. May need a series of VDRLs to follow the titers. Obtain specific cultures for gonorrhea and chlamydia.
         b. Question patient regarding possible exposure, history, or presence of signs and symptoms.
            (1) If negative, assure patient that positive RPR does not necessarily indicate syphilis and await FTA or VDRL.
            (2) If positive, ask patient to come in for physical exam for signs of primary or secondary lesions.
   B. Diagnosis of syphilis at other times.
      1. Indicators that a patient may have syphilis
         a. Signs and symptoms of syphilis
         b. Diagnosis of gonorrhea, chlamydia, or both
         c. Patient expresses concern that she may have an STD.
   C. Treatment
      1. Usual treatment is penicillin because it crosses the placenta. If allergic to penicillin, use erythromycin. It only partially crosses the placenta, so the baby may need treatment after birth.
         a. Early syphilis—primary, secondary, or latent of less than 1 year's duration—must have documented nonreactive RPR or VDRL within the last year. Otherwise, treat as syphilis of more than 1 year's duration:
            (1) Standard treatment: Benzathine Penicillin G, 2.4 million units IM two doses given at 1-week intervals.
            (2) If allergic to penicillin and pregnant or breastfeeding: Erythromycin base (not stearate) 500 mg orally four times a day for 15 days.
         b. Syphilis of more than 1 year's duration
            (1) Standard treatment: Benzathine Penicillin G, 2.4 million units IM three doses given at 1-week intervals.
            (2) If allergic to penicillin and pregnant or breastfeeding: Erythromycin 500 mg orally four times a day for 30 days.
      2. Follow-up VDRL should be repeated monthly while pregnant and at least 3 to 12 months after treatment. Patients with syphilis of

more than 1 year's duration should have a repeat VDRL 24 months after treatment.
3. Patients with documentation of adequate treatment who have a positive VDRL should not be retreated unless there is a fourfold rise in titer.
4. Patient should be told of her diagnosis and how it is acquired and the necessity of completion of treatment and follow-up.
5. Epidemiologic follow-up is needed by the Health Department; it will make every effort to contact the patient's sexual partner(s) and confirm their treatment.

D. The pediatrician or neonatal nurse practitioner, as well as the nursery, need to be notified of the problem at the time of delivery.

THROMBOPHLEBITIS

I. **Definition:** Venous inflammation with thrombus formation
II. **Etiology**
   A. May reflect extension of infection via the veins originating from infected thrombosed veins at the placental site. Extension is either into the pelvic veins (eg, ovarian, renal inferior vena cava) or into the femoral vein from the uterine veins via the iliac veins.
   B. Unknown etiology but is associated with:
      1. Pre-existing varicosities
      2. Pregnancy
      3. Trauma
III. **Clinical Features**
   A. General signs and symptoms
      1. Unexplained elevation of pulse often occurs as first sign.
      2. Repeated severe chills are characteristic.
      3. Extreme swings in temperature, climbing from subnormal to 105°F and then falling precipitously within an hour's time.
      4. Hypotension resulting from bacterial shock.
      5. Small pulmonary emboli causing pleurisy and pneumonia.
   B. Venous thrombosis
      1. Superficial
         a. Slight temperature
         b. Slight pulse elevation
         c. Leg pain
         d. Local heat, extreme tenderness, and redness at site of vein inflammation
      2. Deep
         a. High fever with tachycardia and chills that may be severe
         b. Presence of Homans's sign—when the foot of affected leg is dorsiflexed, there is pain at the site.
         c. Abrupt onset with severe leg pain
         d. Extremity may be discolored, pale, cool, with decrease in pulse pressure below the affected area.
   C. Pulmonary embolism
      1. Most likely with deep venous thrombophlebitis, unlikely with superficial thrombophlebitis
      2. Never massage the leg, it may release a thrombus into the circulation.
III. **Management**
   A. In collaboration with physician
   B. Bed rest
   C. Elevation of the affected extremity

D. Hot packs to the affected extremity
E. Analgesia as needed
F. A cradle for bedclothes if leg is tender to touch
G. Possible anticoagulant and/or antibiotic therapy
H. Consider low dose aspirin daily

NOTES

THYROID DISEASE

I. **Definition:** An abnormality of the thyroid gland, which is the largest endocrine gland. It produces hormones that are vital in maintaining normal growth and metabolism.

II. **Etiology**
   A. The thyroid gland becomes more vascular and enlarges slightly during pregnancy.
   B. Iodine uptake by the thyroid is increased. This change is due to a large increase in serum proteins to which thyroid hormones are bound. The blood level of free, active thyroxine is actually slightly reduced during pregnancy.
   C. The basal metabolic rate increases steadily during pregnancy, but most of the increase is due to the metabolism of the fetus and placenta.

III. **Clinical Features**
   A. Hyperthyroidism
      1. Prominent eyes
      2. Increased appetite and weight loss
      3. Tachycardia
      4. Increased bowel movement, diarrhea
      5. Heat intolerance
      6. Amenorrhea or oligomenorrhea
   B. Hypothyroidism
      1. Fatigue
      2. Constipation
      3. Weight gain not accounted for by excessive food intake
      4. Edema
      5. Hoarse voice
      6. Hair becomes dry and thin
      7. History of abnormal uterine bleeding
      8. History of infertility or amenorrhea

IV. **Differential Diagnosis**
   A. Palpable nodules indicate a focal enlargement; cancer of the thyroid must be ruled out.
   B. Diffuse enlargement or goiter is usually benign but may become obstructive.
   C. Inflammation of the thyroid:
      1. Pain in neck, worse on swallowing
      2. May be transient hyperthyroidism or permanent hypothyroidism

V. **Management**
   A. History
      1. When was last thorough medical evaluation for patient's thyroid condition?

2. Is patient currently on thyroid medication? If so, what type and how much?
3. When was patient last examined by the person who prescribed medication?
- **B.** If thyroid condition is being managed by a physician, patient should be instructed to inform this physician of her current pregnancy and seek a projected plan of thyroid management throughout the pregnancy. Send letter to managing physician.
- **C.** Routinely palpate thyroid on initial physical exam, 6 week postpartum exam, and other times as indicated.
- **D.** Obtain T_3, T_4, T_7, and TSH if any of the following situations exist:
  1. Patient has been on chronic thyroid medication since before pregnancy and is not being currently managed by a physician for her thyroid condition.
  2. Patient gives a history of being on thyroid medicine in the past.
  3. Any abnormality of the thyroid on exam
  4. Signs and/or symptoms of disease

NOTES

TRICHOMONAS VAGINITIS

I. **Definition:** A sexually transmitted infection caused by *Trichomonas*, pear-shaped one-celled protozoa, which are slightly larger than white blood cells, with several flagella that make them extremely motile.

II. **Etiology**
   A. Although usually sexually transmitted, it has been shown to survive for 90 minutes on a wet sponge, suggesting that transmission could occur from a bath, toilet seat, washcloth, or douche equipment.
   B. Although not usually symptomatic in men, they harbor it in their urethra, and can transmit it to women.
   C. May involve the paraurethral Skene's glands and occasionally the lower urinary tract.
   D. Trichomonas prefers a pH higher than that of the normal vagina, and therefore may multiply more rapidly during or immediately following menstruation or during pregnancy.
   E. Trichomonas can carry bacteria to the tubes and cause PID.

III. **Clinical Features**
   A. Signs and symptoms
      1. Fifty percent of affected women may be asymptomatic.
      2. Severe vulvar and vaginal edema, excoriation, itching, burning may be present.
      3. Frothy thin greenish-yellow discharge is characteristic, although the discharge may be thin, white, relatively scanty, and non-frothy.
      4. Red patches on the cervix and vaginal mucosa (the characteristic "strawberry patches") in 10%
      5. Malodorous discharge
      6. Dyspareunia and dysuria are common.
   B. Microscopic examination of wet mount reveals:
      1. The motile colorless pyriform flagellated Trichomonas readily seen in most cases. The specimen must be kept warm to preserve their motility; nonmotile Trichomonas are indistinguishable from white cells.
      2. Numerous white blood cells
      3. Absence of lactobacilli
   C. Apply nitrazene paper to discharge. pH may be 5.5 or more with Trichomonas. Normal pH of 4 to 4.5 virtually rules out Trichomonas.
   D. Trichomonas can occasionally be observed on Pap smears or urinalysis.

IV. **Management**
   A. See Vaginal Discharge Guidelines on page 249 for differential diagnosis.
   B. Avoid treatment in the first trimester of pregnancy.
      1. If symptomatic and need to treat give:
         a. MetroGel vaginal cream at bedtime for 7 days

       b. Betadine vaginal gel
   2. Partner should be treated with Flagyl (metronidazole) 2 gm orally in one dose.
C. In second or third trimester, treat with Flagyl 250 mg orally three times a day for 5 days or 375 mg orally twice a day for 5 days.
   1. The smaller dose over a longer period of time is preferable to a large one-time dose.
   2. The partner(s) should also be treated. Abstinence is urged during the course of treatment to avoid reinfection. Use condoms if abstinence is not carried out.
   3. The patient and her partner should be advised to avoid alcohol during the course of treatment to avoid nausea and vomiting from the Flagyl.
   4. The patient should be warned that monilia vaginitis may develop secondary to Flagyl therapy.
   5. Flagyl is absolutely contraindicated in the first trimester due to potential teratogenic effects.
D. If the patient is not pregnant, she and her partner can be treated with Flagyl, either 250 mg orally three times a day for 5 days, 375 mg orally twice a day for 5 days, or 2 gm orally in a one-time dose.

NOTES

TUBERCULOSIS

I. **Definition:** Tuberculosis (TB) is an acute or chronic infection caused by the bacterium *Mycobacterium tuberculosis*. It is acquired from a person with active TB through airborne transmission.

II. **Incidence**
   A. The incidence of TB in the United States had been declining since the 1900s, but in 1985 the trend reversed. At present, 10 million new cases occur annually, resulting in 3 million deaths.
   B. Recent appearance of strains resistant to multiple anti-TB drugs are cause for concern.

III. **Clinical Features**
   A. Usually asymptomatic at first until lesion is large enough to be visible on radiograph
   B. First signs are fever, general malaise, and weight loss.
   C. Chronic cough more frequent in the morning
   D. Sputum will increase in amount and may be blood-tinged.
   E. Increasing chest pain
   F. TB can become systemic; signs and symptoms will depend on location.

IV. **Management**
   A. Diagnosis
      1. Skin tests are effective 10 weeks after exposure.
         a. Mantoux—a purified protein derivative (PPD) that is injected intradermally in the forearm and read 48 to 72 hours later.
            (1) A test is positive with a 15 mm or more induration.
            (2) It is safe to use in pregnancy.
         b. Tine Test
            (1) Prongs are coated with the PPD.
            (2) 2 mm of induration is considered positive.
         c. False-negative PPDs can occur if:
            (1) The test is given incorrectly.
            (2) The person's immune system is compromised (ie, HIV, malnutrition, corticosteroid use).
            (3) Less than 10 weeks after exposure
         d. False positives often occur with allergies or if the person has been given bacillus Calmette-Guérin (BCG), a live bacterial vaccine often used in third world countries to protect against TB.
      2. Chest radiographs should be done on all positive PPDs and on any negative PPD tests where the patient has symptoms of the disease, or has been exposed to TB.
         a. Use an abdominal shield in pregnancy and wait, if possible, until the second trimester.

b. A radiograph will help distinguish between latent and active TB.
   c. Sputum cultures can be used to confirm active TB.
B. Treatment
   1. Latent TB—there is a 10% chance that latent TB will become active.
      a. Isoniazid hydrochloride (INH) 300 mg orally every day. For 6 months, reduces the incidence of latent disease becoming active.
      b. HIV patients should complete a 12-month course of INH.
      c. Pregnant women need vitamin B_6 25 to 50 mg orally every day to prevent the development of peripheral neuropathy associated with INH.
   2. A patient with active TB should be referred for treatment.
      a. Medications are usually ordered for 6 to 12 months. These may include INH, rifampin, ethambutol, and pyrazinamide.
      b. Sputum should return to negative in 3 to 4 weeks.
   3. Family and contacts need to be tested.
C. Teaching
   1. Need for mask when active TB is present. Cover mouth when coughing. Good hygiene because TB is airborne.
   2. Need to comply with all of the medical treatment for as long as necessary.
   3. Latent TB is not contagious. To prevent it from becoming active, it is important to take daily medicine per recommendation for 6 to 12 months.

NOTES

URINARY TRACT INFECTIONS

I. **Definitions**
   A. Asymptomatic bacteriuria-colony count of more than 100,00 bacteria per ml of urine.
   B. Urethritis: Inflammation of the urethra
   C. Cystitis: Inflammation of the bladder
   D. Pyelonephritis: Inflammation of the kidney

II. **Etiology**
   A. Antepartum: Urinary stasis due to effects of progesterone
      1. Ureteral dilatation
      2. Slowed ureteral peristalsis
      3. Increased pressure from enlarging uterus
   B. Intrapartum
      1. Catheterization secondary to regional anesthesia—while catheterization does not otherwise significantly lead to UTI, the incidence of UTI secondary to catheterization at delivery is 20%.
      2. Trauma and swelling of urethra secondary to use of forceps or other traumatic delivery.
   C. Postpartum
      1. Diuresis after delivery can lead to overdistention and stasis.
      2. Use of oxytocin causes antidiuresis until metabolized then there is a surge of diuresis, which rapidly distends the bladder.
   D. Interconceptionally—may be related to:
      1. Sexual activity. Intercourse can result in introduction of bacteria to the urethra.
      2. Poor hygiene habits
         a. Not washing enough or changing underwear or peripads often enough, thus allowing bacteria near the urethra to multiply.
         b. Wiping from back to front, thus introducing bacteria from the rectum into the urethra.
      3. Health habits such as:
         a. Not emptying the bladder often enough, which results in stasis of urine.
         b. Excessive use of caffeine, which causes urinary irritation and diuresis.
         c. Excessive stress

III. **Clinical Features**
   A. Asymptomatic bacteriuria: no symptoms
   B. Cystitis
      1. Symptoms
         a. Urinary frequency
         b. Urinary urgency

     c. Dysuria
     d. Suprapubic pain
     e. Hematuria
  2. Signs
     a. Bacteriuria-colony count greater than 100,000
     b. Nitrates, a byproduct of bacteria in the urine
     c. WBCs greater than 50/ml or 25 per high power field (HPF) spun urine
     d. RBCs in urine
  C. Pyelonephritis
     1. Fever over 100°F or more with shaking chills
     2. Low back pain
     3. Anorexia, nausea, vomiting
     4. History of UTIs in past
     5. Urinary urgency, frequency, dysuria
     6. CVA tenderness
     7. Suprapubic pain
     8. Bacteria, nitrates, WBCs, RBCs, protein in urine
IV. **Differential Diagnosis**
   A. Urethritis, especially that caused by chlamydia
   B. Vaginitis, vulvitis, or trauma may mimic dysuria.
   C. Frequency may be normal for pregnancy.
V. **Management**
   A. At the initial OB visit, obtain a history of urinary tract infections and a clean-catch urinalysis (CCUA) and urine culture and sensitivity to check for asymptomatic UTI.
      1. If negative history:
         a. And initial negative culture, no further testing is needed unless symptoms develop.
         b. And initial positive culture, treat and repeat urine culture 1 week after treatment and at 28 weeks.
   B. Obtain test of urine at each prenatal visit
      1. If positive for bacteria, nitrates, or blood obtain CCUA.
      2. If more than a trace proteinuria:
         a. Obtain CCUA and recheck.
         b. If still present, rule out pre-eclampsia and pregnancy-induced hypertension (PIH).
         c. If no hypertension, obtain urine C&S to rule out asymptomatic UTI.
         d. If proteinuria is 1+ or greater at two office visits, may wish to do a 24-hour urine for total protein. Consult as necessary.
   C. Any time patient presents with signs and symptoms of cystitis:
      1. Obtain a CCUA and urine culture and sensitivity.

a. If negative in the presence of symptoms, consider GC culture and/or chlamydia culture.
b. If positive, may initiate treatment before results of culture obtained if classic symptoms are present.
2. Check for CVA tenderness.
3. May prescribe Pyridium 100 mg orally three times a day for days to relieve dysuria.

D. Treatment
1. Treat with antibiotics if indicated by results of CCUA and/or urine culture and sensitivity.
   a. Sulfa drugs are most effective.
      (1) They should not be used in the following situations:
         (a) Allergy to sulfa
         (b) After 36 weeks' gestation because sulfa can lead to kernicterus of the newborn
         (c) Patient with G6PD anemia because they can lead to hemolytic anemia.
      (2) If sulfa drugs are used, one choice is Bactrim 500 mg orally twice a day for 7 to 10 days.
   b. Nitrofurantoin (Furadantin, Macrodantin) is also very effective. If used, prescribe 100 mg orally twice a day or 50 mg orally four times a day for 7 days.
   c. Ampicillin 500 mg orally four times a day for 7 to 10 days
   d. Keflex 500 mg orally four times a day for 7 to 10 days
2. Response to antibiotics is usually rapid. Symptoms disappear 1 to 2 days after starting treatment. The patient may feel the infection is gone and discontinue treatment. She should be instructed to take the antibiotic for the full 7 to 10 days to prevent relapse.
3. Warn patient that monilia vaginitis may develop secondary to antibiotic therapy. She should be alert for signs and symptoms.
4. Repeat urine culture 1 week after treatment if patient is pregnant. Cultures should be negative within 24 hours of starting antibiotic therapy.
5. Teach self-help/self-prevention measures.

E. Any time patient presents with signs and symptoms of pyelonephritis:
1. Obtain CCUA, urine culture, CBC
2. Physical exam for costovertebral angle tenderness (CVAT), discomfort over symphysis

F. If patient has UTI twice or more during pregnancy:
1. Consider screening for:
   a. Sickle-cell anemia if patient is African American. Should have been done routinely at initial OB visit.
   b. G6PD anemia if patient is African American, Asian, or of Mediterranean descent
   c. Diabetes

2. May need tests of kidney function, such as blood urea nitrogen (BUN), creatinine, 24-hour urinary creatinine clearance, total protein
3. Prophylactic prevention with Macrodantin 50 to 100 mg orally every day
4. May need urology consult

G. Self-help measures:
1. Drink at least 8 to 10 glasses of liquid daily to encourage adequate kidney function and prevent urinary stasis.
2. Avoid caffeine, which is irritating to the urinary system and acts as a diuretic. Excess vitamin C is also an irritant.
3. Use proper perineal hygiene to prevent urethral contamination from rectal bacteria.
4. Urinate frequently throughout the day to prevent urinary stasis.
5. Urinate immediately after intercourse to wash away bacteria that may have been moved to the urethra.

NOTES

VACCINATIONS

I. **Live Virus**

   Vaccination with live virus is never recommended in pregnancy. Killed virus may be considered if risk of disease outweighs the risk of exposure to vaccination during pregnancy.

II. **Specific Types of Vaccination**

   A. Flu vaccine
   1. The CDC recommends flu vaccinations for women who have an underlying high-risk condition.
   2. Vaccine should be avoided until the second or third trimester if at all possible.

   B. Rubella vaccine—see Rubella Guidelines on page 222.
   1. Not recommended during pregnancy or sooner than 3 months before conception due to possible teratogenic effects.
   2. If patient is rubella negative, she should be vaccinated in the immediate postpartum period to prevent possible exposure and resultant teratogenic effects in subsequent pregnancy.
   3. Informed consent should be obtained before vaccination. About 10% to 12% develop transient arthritis. Risks to others in her environment are minimal.

   C. Hepatitis vaccine (Heptovax)—see Hepatitis Guidelines on page 147.
   1. Consists of killed virus, so should logically be safe in pregnancy, but has not been widely used. Weigh potential risk of hepatitis versus benefits.

NOTES

VAGINAL DISCHARGE

I. **Incidence:** The most frequent complaint of women presenting for gynecologic care.
II. **Etiology and Management**
   A. Extravaginal disease simulating vaginal discharge
      1. Vulvar and/or perineal lesions
         a. Syphilis chancre
         b. Chancroid
         c. Herpes
         d. Condylomata
         e. Cancer
         f. Miscellaneous—psoriasis, dermatitis, parasitic infestations, etc.
      2. Bartholinitis/Bartholin's cyst
      3. Proctitis
      4. Vaginal fistulae
   B. Physiologic discharge—a normal discharge, which is cervical in origin
      1. Most apparent in high estrogen states
         a. At the time of ovulation
         b. During pregnancy
         c. During oral contraceptive use
      2. Changes in cervical mucous during the menstrual cycle
         a. Just after menses, hormone levels are low, causing mucous to be scant and sticky.
         b. As estrogen increases, mucous increases in amount and becomes thinner.
         c. At midcycle, the mucous is clear, slippery, and stretchy, like raw egg white. This mucous heralds ovulation and the fertile period.
         d. After ovulation, progesterone dominates, making the mucous decreased in amount, sticky, and cloudy.
   C. Noninfectious vaginal discharge
      1. Local irritation or allergic response
         a. Usual causative agents
            (1) Douche chemical
            (2) Feminine hygiene products
            (3) Sexual aid products
            (4) Contraceptive creams, foams, jellies (nonoxynol 9)
         b. Diagnosis
            (1) Confirmed by finding large numbers of eosinophils in the discharge via wet prep
            (2) Clears up when use of the offending agent is stopped

2. Foreign object in the vagina
   a. Usual causative agents—A forgotten tampon or diaphragm
   b. Pathology
      (1) Discharge
         (a) Often scanty but may be purulent, brown-tinged, or frankly bloody
         (b) May have offensive odor
      (2) May be signs of infection
   c. Management
      (1) Examiner should double-glove the examining hand, remove the foreign object, fold the top glove of the examining hand over the object, tie a knot in the end, and discard.
      (2) If there are signs of significant irritation or infection, order vaginal cream or an oral antibiotic.
3. Atrophic vaginitis
   a. Caused by a low estrogen state
      (1) Prepuberty
      (2) Lactation
      (3) Postmenopause
   b. High pH of vagina changes the normal flora.
   c. Vaginal mucosa is thin and therefore susceptible to infection and trauma.
   d. Symptoms
      (1) Dyspareunia
      (2) Postcoital spotting
      (3) Vulvar irritation
   e. Wet prep reveals
      (1) Immature epithelial cells
      (2) Large numbers of WBCs
   f. Treatment
      (1) Rule out secondary infection
      (2) Topical estrogen cream works well. Estrace 0.1% or premarin 0.625 mg/gram at bedtime for 1 week, four times a day for 1 week, twice a week for 2 weeks, then a maintenance dose of 1 to 2 days per week.
4. Cervicitis: An infection of the endocervix
   a. Causes 30% of all vaginal discharge
   b. Clinical picture
      (1) Mucopurulent discharge coming from os
      (2) Cervix inflamed, friable, bleeding, or edematous.
   c. Symptoms
      (1) Mucopurulent discharge
      (2) Intermenstrual or postcoital spotting

d. Causes
   (1) STDs
   (2) Cervical cap
   (3) Cancer may be cause or secondary effect
5. Neoplasia—discharge starts gradually, similar to that seen in foreign body irritation. Consult.

D. Infectious vaginal discharge
1. *Trichomonas vaginalis*—see Trichomonas vaginitis on page 240. Discharge is frothy, thin, yellow-green/gray, irritating, malodorous.
2. *Candida albicans*—see Monilia vaginitis on page 182. Discharge is cheesy, curdy, yellow-white, irritating, may smell yeasty.
3. *Gardnerella*—see Gardnerella vaginitis on page 253. Discharge is minimal, creamy, yellow/gray, malodorous.
4. *Neisseria gonorrhoeae*—see Gonorrhea on page 137. May be no discharge, or may be green or yellow-green, irritating.
5. *Treponema pallidum*—see Syphilis on page 232. Not usually a discharge, although chancres or condylomata may be weepy or infected.
6. *Herpes virus*—see Herpes Simplex on page 152. May be grayish exudate or thin discharge from weepy lesions or superinfection.
7. *Chlamydia*—see Chlamydia guidelines on page 96. May be no discharge or may be mucopurulent, foul smelling.

III. Clinical Features
A. History
1. Age
   a. Women in sexually active years most likely to present with STDs.
   b. Older women most likely to have neoplasms, although young women get them too.
   c. Any vaginal discharge is unlikely in a prepubescent girl and warrants vigorous workup.
2. Mode and time of onset
   a. A woman who can say exactly which day her discharge began is likely to have an infection.
   b. Relationship to menstrual cycle
      (1) Onset of discharge in the premenstrual period may indicate monilia vaginitis.
      (2) Discharge beginning at the time of the menses is likely to be trichomonas vaginitis or gonorrhea.
      (3) Discharge at midcycle and up to a week after may be physiological
3. Presence of other diseases
   a. Diabetes and hypoparathyroidism are associated with an increased frequency of monilia vaginitis.

b. Impaired resistance to infection, such as leukemia, chronic renal or hepatic disease, or collagen vascular disease, can predispose to vaginitis.
4. Contraceptive history
   a. Oral contraceptives may predispose to monilia.
   b. IUD may predispose to PID.
   c. Cervical cap may cause cervical ulcer/local cervicitis.
   d. Spermicides may cause chemical irritation and/or allergy.
5. History of current and prior medications
   a. Locally applied chemicals can cause vaginitis
   b. Antibiotics, including Flagyl, steroids, and oral contraceptives can lead to candida infection.
   c. Low-dose or broad-spectrum antibiotics can mask tests for gonorrhea and syphilis and result in an antibiotic-resistant strain.
6. Sexual history—ask: "Do you have reason to suspect that you may have a sexually transmitted disease?"
   a. Dates and treatment of previous conditions
   b. Previous condition not resolved or is recurring
   c. New sexual partners, number of partners, and whether steady or casual
7. Hygiene habits may be causing local irritation.
   a. Poor hygiene, may be secondary to obesity
   b. Frequent use of douches, chemical sprays, and other hygiene products

B. Physical exam
1. Inspect external genitalia for:
   a. Erythema, edema, excoriation
   b. Lesions—note whether draining or not.
   c. Presence of discharge at the introitus
   d. Discharge from Bartholin's or paraurethral Skene's glands; purulent discharge indicative of gonorrhea
2. Palpate for inguinal lymphadenopathy, which would indicate an infectious process as in syphilis or herpes
3. Speculum exam:
   a. Inspect vaginal walls and cervix for irritation, lesions, and discharge.
      (1) Monilia: White patches on vaginal and/or cervical mucosa
      (2) Trichomonas: Red, inflamed, ``strawberry patches'' appearance of vaginal and/or cervical mucosa
      (3) Herpes: Cervicitis usually present only in primary episodes, ulcers usually only in endocervix
   b. If indicated, gather specimens.
      (1) Swab for wet prep.

    (2) Cultures:
        (a) General culture of discharge can diagnose bacterial infections, such as gardnerella, beta-strep, other bacteria.
        (b) GC/chlamydia culture of cervix and lesions
        (c) Herpes culture of cervix and lesions
        (d) Chlamydia culture
    (3) Pap smear will report infections, cell changes.
4. Bimanual exam
    a. Palpate cervix for cervical motion tenderness—indicative of PID, gonorrhea.
    b. Palpate uterus, adnexa
        (1) Check for:
            (a) Masses
            (b) Enlargement
            (c) Abnormal shape, consistency, position
            (d) Tenderness

IV. Management
A. Labwork
    1. Evaluate wet prep.
        a. Positive whiff test is indicative of bacterial vaginosis (BV) (Gardnerella)
        b. Clue cells are indicative of BV.
        c. Trichomonads are diagnostic of Trichomonas vaginitis.
        d. Filaments with budding spores and/or pseudo hyphae are diagnostic of monilia vaginitis.
        e. Immature cells and numerous WBCs are indicative of infection and possible atrophic vaginitis.
        f. Numerous eosinophils are indicative of allergic response.
        g. Numerous Döderlein's bacilli (lactobacilli) are indicative of physiologic discharge.
    2. Normal pH of vaginal discharge is 4.5 plus or minus 0.5.
        a. Under 4.5 is indicative of a high estrogen state, such as pregnancy.
        b. Over 5 is indicative of:
            (1) Low estrogen state as in atrophic vaginitis
            (2) Monilia, trichomonas, or gardnerella vaginitis
    3. Blood work
        a. Rapid plasma reagent (RPR) or fluorescent treponema antibody (FTA) if clinical picture suggestive of herpes
        b. Antibody titers if primary herpes
        c. CBC with differential if signs of systemic infection, PID
    4. Pap smear can diagnose:
        a. Dysplasia or carcinoma

       b. Monilia vaginitis
       c. Gardnerella vaginitis
       d. Herpes simplex
       e. Human papillomavirus (HPV)
       f. May be suggestive of Trichomonas vaginitis or chlamydia, but do not treat until specific tests are done to confirm or rule out diagnosis.

B. Treatment
   1. Diagnose according to history, physical exam, and labwork.
   2. Manage and treat according to specific guidelines.
   3. General patient teaching
       a. Educate regarding characteristics of normal vaginal discharge.
       b. Avoid use of irritating products.
       c. Practice good hygiene.
       d. Monilia vaginitis is a common superinfection when broad-spectrum antibiotics are taken; use preventative treatment measures.
       e. With each new partner or with multiple partners, the risk for vaginal infection increases.
       f. With active symptoms of infection, intercourse should be avoided until treatment of infection.
       g. If the infection is sexually transmitted, the partner(s) may need to be treated.
       h. While undergoing treatment, avoid intercourse or use condoms if the infection could be sexually transmitted.
       i. Examination and laboratory tests are necessary for diagnosis.
       j. Patient must use all the medication prescribed, not just until the symptoms are gone.
       k. A vaginal infection may cause an abnormal Pap smear.
       l. A follow-up examination to test for cure may be necessary.

IV

Drug Index

This drug index provides a quick reference to the commonly used drugs suggested in the other chapters. The description of each drug includes the generic name, class of drug, pregnancy category, indications, contraindications, dosages, side effects, and drug interactions. It is especially important, when caring for pregnant women, to be aware of the effects of a drug on the fetus and on the baby when the patient is lactating. To that end, each drug described has a classification indicating safety in pregnancy. An explanation of those classifications is seen below.

Category A: Well-controlled human studies have not disclosed any fetal risks.

Category B: Animal studies have not disclosed any fetal risk; or suggested some risk which is not confirmed in controlled studies in women; or there are no adequate studies in women.

Category C: Animal studies reveal adverse fetal effects; there are no adequate controlled studies in women.

Category D: Some fetal risk. Benefits may outweigh risk (eg, life-threatening illness, no safer effective drug available). Patient should be warned.

Category X: Fetal abnormalities in animal and human studies. Risk does not outweigh benefit. **Contraindicated in pregnancy.**

ACTIFED

TRIPROLIDINE HCL & PSEUDOEPHEDRINE HCL

Drug classes: Antihistamine, sympathomimetic

Pregnancy Category B

Indications:
- Rhinorrhea
- Congestion

Adults: One tablet orally every 4 to 6 hours; maximum four doses a day. Also 12-hour capsules: One capsule every 12 hours.

Contraindications: During or within 14 days of monoamine oxidase inhibitors, severe hypertension or coronary artery disease, gastrointestinal or urinary obstruction

Precautions: Thyroid disease, diabetes

Interactions: Hypertensive crisis with monoamine oxidase inhibitors, β-blockers may increase the pressor effects of sympathomimetics. Alcohol, other central nervous system depressants potentiated.

Adverse reactions: Drowsiness, anticholinergic effects, gastrointestinal upset, dizziness, anxiety, weakness, insomnia, thickening of bronchial secretions, hypotension, respiratory depression or difficulty, palpitations

How supplied: Tablets, 12-hour capsules, syrup—4 ounce, pint

NOTES

ACYCLOVIR

ZOVIRAX

Drug classes: Antiviral, purine nucleoside analogue
Pregnancy Category C

Indications:
- Genital herpes
- Herpes zoster (shingles)
- Varicella (chickenpox)

Adults: Genital herpes: Initial 400 mg twice to four times a day for 10 to 14 days, recurring 400 twice a day 5 to 7 days. Chronic: 400 mg daily up to 12 months. Herpes zoster: 800 mg every 4 hours (maximum: 5 times a day) for 7 to 10 days. Varicella: Initiate at earliest sign, 20 mg/kg four times daily for 5 days; maximum: 800 mg/dose.

Contraindications: Allergy to Acyclovir, renal disease, seizures, congestive heart failure, pregnancy, lactation

Interactions: Probenecid decreases urinary excretion of acyclovir.

Adverse reactions: Nausea, vomiting, headache, central nervous system disturbances, diarrhea, vertigo, arthralgia, rash, malaise, fatigue, viral resistance

How supplied: Tablets 200, 400 mg

AMOXICILLIN

TRIMOX, AMOXIL

Drug class: Broad-spectrum penicillin
Pregnancy Category B

Indications:
- Amoxicillin-sensitive infections including ear, respiratory or genitourinary tract, skin, soft tissue, acute uncomplicated gonorrhea

Adults: 250 to 500 mg orally every 8 hours. Gonorrhea: 3 g once.

Contraindications: Contraindicated in the presence of allergies to penicillins, cephalosporins, or other allergens. Use caution in the presence of renal disorders, lactation.

Precautions: Cephalosporin or other allergy; not recommended. Monitor blood, renal, and liver function in long-term use. Continue therapy for 2 to 3 days after symptoms improve. Lactation.

Interactions Potentiated by probenecid

Adverse reactions: Superinfection, anaphylaxis, urticaria, gastrointestinal upset, blood dyscrasias, hyperactivity

How supplied Capsules: 250, 500 mg; chewables: 125, 250 mg

Group B Strept: 250-500 mg bid x 7

AMPICILLIN

OMNIPEN, PRINCIPEN

Drug class: Broad-spectrum penicillin

Pregnancy Category B

Indications:
- Amoxicillin-sensitive infections

Adults: 250 to 500 mg orally four times a day; gonorrhea: 3.5 g with 1 g probenecid

Contraindications: Contraindicated in the presence of allergies to penicillins, cephalosporins, or other allergens. Use caution in the presence of renal disorders.

Precautions: Allergy to cephalosporin, imipenem; mononucleosis; not recommended

Monitor blood, renal, and liver function in long-term use. Continue therapy for 2 to 3 days after symptoms improve.

Interactions: Potentiated by probenecid

Adverse reactions Superinfection, anaphylaxis, urticaria, gastrointestinal upset, blood dyscrasias, hyperactivity

How supplied: Capsules 100, 500 mg; chewables: 125, 250 mg; suspension: 80, 100, 180 ml; drops 50 mg/ml

NOTES

ASPIRIN

BAYER, ECOTRIN, EMPIRIN

Drug classes: Antipyretic, analgesic, anti-inflammatory, antirheumatic, antiplatelet, salicylate, nonsteroidal anti-inflammatory drug

Pregnancy Category D

Indications:
- Mild to moderate pain
- Fever

Adults: 325 to 650 mg orally every 4 hours as needed; maximum: 12 tablets daily

Contraindications: Nonsteroidal anti-inflammatory drug allergy; third trimester pregnancy

Precautions: History of asthma or peptic ulcer, impaired renal or hepatic function, bleeding disorders, erosive gastritis, diabetes, gout. Monitor blood pressure, blood urea nitrogen, uric acid levels. Pregnancy, lactation.

Interactions: Para-aminobenzoic acid may increase serum levels. May potentiate anticoagulants, hypoglycemics, methotrexate. Urinary alkalinizers, antacids, corticosteroids may increase excretions. May antagonize uricosurics, spironolactone.

Adverse reactions: Gastric upset, prolonged bleeding time, asthma, rhinitis, urticaria, anaphylaxis, salicylism.

How supplied: Varies with manufacturer

NOTES

AZT

(ZIDOVUDINE) RETROVIR

Drug class: Antiviral

Pregnancy Category C

Indications:

- Some patients with human immunodeficiency virus infection (and advanced AIDS-related complex) and a history of cytologically confirmed *Pneumocystis carinii* pneumonia or an absolute CD4 (T4 helper/inducer) lymphocyte count of less than $200/mm^3$
- Human immunodeficiency virus patients with evidence of impaired immunity (CD, cell count of $<500/mm^3$)
- When given during pregnancy, will decrease transfer of infection to fetus.

Adults: Symptomatic human immunodeficiency virus. Infection: Initially 200 mg every 4 hours (2.9 mg/kg every four hours) orally, around the clock. Monitor hematologic indices every 2 weeks. If anemia is significant, (hemoglobin <7.5 g/dl, reduction of >25%) or reduction of granulocytes more than 50% below baseline, dose interruption is necessary until evidence of bone marrow recovery is shown. If less severe bone marrow depression occurs, dosage reduction may be adequate; or 1 to 2 mg/kg every 4 hours intravenously.

Asymptomatic human immunodeficiency virus infection: 100 mg every 4 hours orally while awake (500 mg/d)

Contraindications: Presence of life-threatening allergy to any component, lactation. Caution in the presence of compromised bone marrow, impaired renal or hepatic function

Adverse reactions: Headache, asthenia, nausea, gastrointestinal pain, diarrhea, agranulocytopenia, fever

How supplied: Capsules 100 mg or intravenous

NOTES

BELLERGAL-S

Drug classes: Barbiturate, ergot alkaloid, anticholinergic
Pregnancy Category X

Indications:
- Menopausal disorders with hot flushes, sweats, restlessness, or insomnia

Adults: 1 tablet twice daily

Contraindications: Coronary or peripheral vascular disease, hypertension, impaired hepatic or renal function, glaucoma. Paradoxical reactions to phenobarbital. Pregnancy, lactation.

Precautions: Gastrointestinal problems, myasthenia gravis, asthma

Interactions: Avoid other vasoconstrictors (eg, dopamine). Concomitant antacids may inhibit absorption. May antagonize anticoagulants. Monitor patients on concomitant β-blockers. Additive anticholinergic effects with tricyclic antidepressants.

Adverse reactions: Drowsiness, nausea, vomiting, local edema, itching, vasoconstrictive complications, tachycardia or bradycardia, pares, anticholinergic effects, paradoxical excitement.

How supplied: Tablets

NOTES

BENADRYL

DIPHENHYDRAMINE HCL

Drug class: Antihistamine

Pregnancy Category B in Third Trimester

Indications:
- Allergic and vasomotor rhinitis, conjunctivitis, pruritus, reactions to blood
- Adjunct in anaphylaxis
- Sleep aid

Adults: 25 to 50 mg orally every 4 to 6 hours; maximum: 300 mg daily. 25 to 50 mg intramuscular every 4 to 6 hours

Contraindications: Contraindicated in the presence of allergy to any antihistamines. Lactation.

Precautions: Asthma and lower respiratory disorders. Glaucoma, hyperthyroidism, hypertension, and cardiovascular disease. Gastrointestinal or urinary obstruction.

Interactions: Potentiates central nervous system depression with alcohol, other central nervous system depressants. Potentiates anticholinergic effects with monoamine oxidase inhibitors.

Adverse reactions: Drowsiness, dizziness, anticholinergic effects, gastritis, paradoxical, excitement, blood dyscrasias, hypotension

How supplied: Capsules: 25, 50 mg; elixir: 12.5 mg/5 ml intramuscular, intravenous 10, 50 mg/ml

BETAMETHASONE DIPROPIONATE

CELESTONE SOLUSPAN

Drug classes: Corticosteroid, glucocorticoid, and hormonal agent

Pregnancy Category C

Indications:
- Maturation of fetal lungs in premature labor

Adults: 12.5 mg intramuscular. Repeat in 24 hours. May be repeated 1 week later.

Contraindications: Not currently approved by the Food and Drug Administration for premature labor. DO NOT give to patients taking anticonvulsant drugs. Allergy to drug.

Adverse reactions: Burning, itching, irritation at injection site, sweating, tachycardia

How supplied: intramuscular 12.5 mg/ml

BICILLIN LONG-ACTING

PENICILLIN G BENZATHINE

Drug class: Antibiotic

Pregnancy Category B

Indications:

- Bactericidal

Adults: Group A streptococcal upper respiratory: 1.2 million units IM in a single dose

Syphilis or less than 1 year's duration: 2.4 million units IM in a single dose

Syphilis of more than 1 year's duration: 2.4 million units IM weekly for 3 successive weeks.

Contraindications: NEVER give intravenously; inadvertent intravenous administration has caused cardiac arrest and death. Use cautiously in patients with other drug allergies, especially to cephalosporins.

Interactions: Potentiated by probenecid

Adverse reactions: Anaphylaxis, seizures, nausea, hemolytic anemia, exfoliative dermatitis

How supplied: Injection: 300,000 or 600,000 units/ml

NOTES

CHOLESTYRAMINE

QUESTRAN LIGHT

Drug class: Bile acid sequestrant

Indications:
- Hypercholesterolemia alone with hypertriglyceridemia resistant to dietary management for the reduction in risk of coronary heart disease.
- Pruritus due to partial biliary obstruction, pregnancy induced.

Adults: Initially 1 packet or scoop mixed with fluid or food one to two times daily. Maintenance: Two to four packets or scoops divided into two doses; maximum: six packets or scoops daily. Increase at 4-week intervals as needed.

Contraindications: Complete biliary obstruction. Lactation.

Precautions: Obtain baseline serum cholesterol, low-density lipoprotein (LDL)-C, triglycerides, and monitor during therapy. May need vitamins A, D, K, and folic acid supplementation with long-term therapy. Exclude secondary causes of hypercholesterolemia. Favorable trend in cholesterol reduction usually occurs within 1 month; continue therapy to sustain reduction. Phenylketonuria; constipation; hemorrhoids.

Interactions: Inhibits absorption of phenylbutazone, warfarin, chlorothiazide, propranolol, tetracycline, penicillin G, phenobarbital, thyroid drugs, digitalis, many others; give other drugs 1 to 2 hours before or 4 to 6 hours after.

Adverse reactions: Constipation, aggravation of hemorrhoids, gastrointestinal disturbances, vitamins A, D, K, or folic acid deficiencies, rash

How supplied: Light 5 g packet-60; 9 g packet-60; 210 g can—1 (with scoop)

CHROMAGEN

Drug class: Hematinics

Indications:
- Iron deficiency

Adults: One capsule orally daily

Contraindications: Hemochromatosis; hemosiderosis

Precautions: Hepatitis, pancreatitis, achlorhydria, peptic ulcer or gastrointestinal inflammation. Monitor hematocrit.

Interactions: Inhibits tetracycline absorption. Antacids inhibit iron absorption.

Adverse reactions: Nausea, rash, vomiting, diarrhea, black stools, flushing

How supplied: Capsules

CLEOCIN/CLEOCIN VAGINAL

CLINDAMYCIN HYDROCHLORIDE

Drug class: Lincosamide antibiotic

Pregnancy Category B

Indications:
- Systematic administrations: serious infections caused by susceptible strains of anaerobes, streptococci, staphylococci, pneumococci
- Reserve use for penicillin-allergic patients
- Treatment of acne vulgaris
- Treatment of bacterial vaginosis

Contraindications: Allergy to clindamycin or history of asthma, tartrazine; hepatic or renal dysfunction; lactation

Adults: 150 to 300 mg orally every 6 hours, up to 300 to 450 mg every 6 hours in more severe infections

For vaginal preparation: one 100 mg clindamycin phosphate preparation intravaginally at bedtime for 7 consecutive days.

Adverse reactions: Systematic administration: nausea, vomiting, diarrhea, abdominal pain, esophagitis, anorexia, and rash. Vaginal preparation: Cervicitis, vaginitis, contact dermitis, dryness.

How supplied: Tablets 75, 150, 300 mg; intravenous and injection: 150, 300 mg/ml; cream

NOTES

CLIMARA

ESTRADIOL

Drug class: Hormone/estrogen
Pregnancy Category X

Indications:
- Estrogen replacement therapy
- Moderate to severe vasomotor symptoms of menopause
- Vulvar or vaginal atrophy

Adults: One 0.1 mg/d patch applied once per week to trunk (avoid breasts and waistline)

Contraindications: Undiagnosed abnormal genital bleeding. Thromboembolic disorders. Breast or estrogen-dependent carcinoma.

Precautions: Familial hyperlipoproteinemia; cardiovascular disease; hepatic, renal, or cardiac insufficiency; asthma; epilepsy; migraine; endometriosis; depression; gallbladder disease. Bone disease associated with hypercalcemia. Uterine leiomyomatas, diabetes, thromboembolic disease. Discontinue if hypertension or jaundice occurs.

Adverse reactions: Increased risk of endometrial cancer or hyperplasia, gallbladder disease, thromboembolic disorders, hepatic tumors, fluid retention, breakthrough bleeding, mastodynia, nausea, abdominal cramps, headache, migraine, dizziness, increased size of uterine fibromyomata, irritation at application site.

How supplied: Patch: 0.05 mg, 0.1 mg

COLACE

DOCUSATE

Drug class: Laxative
Pregnancy Category C

Indications:
- Short-term relief of constipation

Adults: 50 to 240 mg orally every every day, twice a day

Contraindications: Third trimester of pregnancy. Acute abdominal disorders: appendicitis, diverticulitis, and ulcerative colitis.

Adverse reactions: Excessive bowel activity, perianal irritation, abdominal cramps, weakness, dizziness, and electrolyte imbalance

How supplied: Tablets 50, 100, 240, 300 mg

DARVOCET-N 100

PROPOXYPHENE NAPSYLATE 100 MG WITH ACETAMINOPHEN 650 MG

Drug class: Opioid

Pregnancy Category C

Indications:
- Mild to moderate pain

Adults: 1 tablet orally every 4 hours as necessary

Contraindications: Suicidal or addiction-prone patients

Interactions: Potentiated with alcohol central nervous system depressants

Adverse reactions: Dizziness, sedation, nausea, vomiting, constipation, rash; respiratory depression

How supplied: Capsules, tablets

DEMEROL

MEPERIDINE

Drug class: Opioid

Pregnancy Category C

Indications:
- Moderate to severe pain

Adults: Pain: 50 mg orally, 50 to 100 mg intramuscular or subcutaneous every 3 to 4 hours as necessary. 25 to 50 mg intravenous every 3 to 4 hours as necessary

Contraindications: Within 14 days of monoamine oxidase inhibitors. Lactation.

Precautions: Increased intracranial pressure; acute abdomen; convulsive disorders; impaired respiratory, renal, hepatic, thyroid, or adrenocortical function; supraventricular tachycardias; drug abusers.

Interactions: Monoamine oxidase inhibitors (toxicity, may be fatal). Potentiation with alcohol, central nervous system depressants, phenothiazines, tricyclics.

Adverse reactions: High abuse potential, sedation, dizziness, sweating, dry mouth, nausea, vomiting, constipation, urinary retention, hypotension, rash; convulsions with large doses; respiratory depression

How supplied: Tablets 25 to 50 mg; injection: 1 ml syrup 25, 50, 75, 100 mg/ml

DEPO-PROVERA

MEDROXYPROGESTERONE ACETATE

Drug classes: Progestogen, progesterone derivative

Pregnancy Category X

Indications:
- Injectable contraception

Adults: 150 mg intramuscular every 12 weeks. Dosage adjustment for body weight not necessary.

Contraindications: Undiagnosed vaginal bleeding; thromboembolic disorders; cerebrovascular disease; hepatic dysfunction; lactation.

Precautions: Asthma; epilepsy; migraine; diabetes; cardiac or renal dysfunction; depression. Discontinue if jaundice, visual disturbances, migraine, or thrombotic disorders occur.

Interactions: May be antagonized by aminoglutethimide

Adverse reactions: Irregular bleeding; edema; weight or cervical changes; cholestatic jaundice; thromboembolic events; depression; pyrexia; insomnia; nausea; somnolence; breast tenderness; galactorrhea; acne; hirsutism; alopecia; rash.

How supplied: Injection 100, 400 mg/ml

DIFLUCAN

FLUCONAZOLE

Drug class: Antifungal

Pregnancy Category B

Indications:
- Candidiasis

Adults: 150 mg orally in a single dose, repeat in 4 to 5 days if condition not completely resolved. 200 to 400 mg orally first day, followed by 100 to 200 every day for 2 weeks for oropharyngeal and systemic candidiasis respectively.

Contraindications: History of regional enteritis, antibiotic associated or ulcerative colitis

Precautions: Lactation

Adverse reactions: Headache, nausea, vomiting, diarrhea, skin rash

How supplied: Tablets 50, 100, 150, 200 mg

DOXYCYCLINE

VIBRAMYCIN

Drug class: Antibiotic
Pregnancy Category D
Indications:
- Pelvic inflammatory disease
- Sexually transmitted diseases when penicillin is contraindicated
- Traveler's diarrhea prophylaxis

Adults: 100 mg orally twice a day for 7 to 10 days. Traveler's diarrhea prophylaxis: 100 mg orally every day. Begin 2 to 3 days before trip

Contraindications: Allergy to tetracyclines; pregnancy; lactation

Precautions: Monitor blood, renal, and liver function in long-term use; sunlight or ultraviolet light

Interactions: Antacids, iron, zinc, calcium, magnesium, urinary alkalinizers reduce absorption. Monitor prothrombin time with oral anticoagulants.

Adverse reactions: Superinfection, photosensitivity, gastrointestinal upset, enterocolitis, rash, blood dyscrasias, hepatotoxicity

How supplied: Capsules 50, 100 mg

EMETROL

Drug class: Phosphorylated carbohydrate
Indications:
- Nausea and vomiting

Adults: 15 to 30 ml orally at 15-minute intervals as needed.

Precautions: Do not dilute or permit oral fluids immediately before or for 15 minutes after dosage. Diabetes.

How supplied: Syrup—4 oz, 8 oz, pint

ENTEX/ENTEX LA

Drug classes: Sympathomimetic and expectorant
Pregnancy Category C

Indications:
- Nasal congestion associated with sinusitis, bronchitis

Adults: Entex: 1 tablet orally every 6 hours—best with food. Entex LA: 1 tablet every 12 hours. DO NOT crush or chew.
Contraindications: Severe hypertension, coronary artery disease. Within 14 days of monoamine oxidase inhibitors.
Precautions: Hypertension; diabetes; cardiovascular disease; glaucoma; elderly; hyperthyroidism.
Interactions: Hypertensive crisis with monoamine oxidase inhibitors. β-blockers may increase the pressor effects of sympathomimetics. Antihypertensives, antagonized.
Adverse reactions: Headaches, nervousness, dizziness, insomnia, convulsions, central nervous system depression, tachycardia, palpitations, urinary retention, gastrointestinal upset.
How supplied: Capsules

EPINEPHRINE

ADRENALIN

Drug classes: Adrenergic bronchodilator and vasopressor
Pregnancy Category C

Indications:
- Anaphylaxis, cardiac arrest, and prolongation of local anesthetic effect.

Adults: Anaphylaxis: 0.1 to 0.5 ml of 1:1,000 subcutaneous or intramuscular; repeat every 10 to 15 minutes as necessary, or 0.1 to 0.25 ml of 1:1,000 intravenous. Cardiac arrest: 0.5 to 1 mg intravenous or endotracheally. May give doses up to 5 mg, especially in patients who do not respond to usual intravenous doses. Maintenance infusion: 1 to 4 µg/min. Local anesthetic effect: 1:500,000 to 1:50,000 mixed with local anesthetic.
Contraindications: Contraindicated in patients with glaucoma; shock; organic brain damage; cardiac dilatation; coronary insufficiency; and during labor. Patients in labor.
Interactions: α-blockers may cause hypotension. β-blockers may cause vasoconstriction and reflex bradycardia.
Adverse reactions: Palpitations; tachycardia; nervousness; and headache; apnea; hypertension; tachyarrhythmias; ventricular fibrillation; cerebrovascular accident.
How supplied: Injection—various strengths

ERYTHROMYCIN, E.E.S., E-MYCIN

ERYTHROMYCIN ETHYLSUCCINATE

Drug class: Macrolide antibiotic

Pregnancy Category B

Indications:

- Susceptible infections including respiratory, skin and soft tissue, genitourinary
- Sexually transmitted diseases: chlamydia, *N. gonorrhoeae*, syphilis

Adults: 250 to 500 mg orally every 6 hours, 1 hour before meals; maximum: 4 g daily for 7 to 10 days. Gonorrhea: 500 mg orally for 3 days 250 mg (base stearate) or 400 mg orally (ethylsuccinate) every 6 hours for 7 days. Chlamydia: 500 mg orally every 6 hours for 7 days. Syphilis: 20 g orally in divided doses over 15 days (base, estolate, stearate).

Contraindications: Allergic to medication. Irritable bowel syndrome, colitis, bowel diseases

Precautions: Hepatic dysfunction

Interactions: May potentiate carbamazepine, methylprednisolone, cyclosporine, digoxin, theophylline, warfarin, ergotamine, terfenadine, triazolam, others.

Adverse reactions: Hepatotoxicity, superinfection, gastrointestinal upset, rash, reversible hearing loss

How supplied: Capsules: 250, 500 mg; cream: 42.5 g

NOTES

ESTRACE/ESTRADIOL 0.01% VAGINAL CREAM

ESTRADIOL/TARTRAZINE

Drug class: Hormone/estrogen

Pregnancy Category X

Indications:
- Moderate to severe vasomotor symptoms associated with menopause
- Vulvular or vaginal atrophy
- Osteoporosis prevention

Adults: 1 to 2 mg orally daily, cyclically. Vaginally every day for 1 week, every other day for 1 week, maintenance dose: one to two times a week

Contraindications: Breast or estrogen-dependent carcinoma; undiagnosed abnormal genital bleeding; thrombophlebitis; thromboembolic disorders or history of associated with previous estrogen use.

Precautions: Increased risk of endometrial carcinoma. If used in a patient with a uterus, a progesterone product will counter this effect. Impaired renal, hepatic, or cardiac function. Immobilized patients; epilepsy; migraine; asthma; diabetes; depression.

Adverse reactions: Breast tenderness and enlargement, uterine bleeding, dysmenorrhea, amenorrhea, vaginal candidiasis, gastrointestinal upset, depression, endometrial carcinoma, gallbladder or thromboembolic disease, hepatic carcinoma, skin changes.

How supplied: Tablets 1, 2 mg

NOTES

ESTRADERM TRANSDERMAL PATCH

ESTRADIOL

Drug class: Hormone/estrogen

Pregnancy Category X

Indications:
- Atrophic vaginitis
- Moderate to severe vasomotor symptoms of menopause
- Postmenopausal osteoporosis prophylaxis

Adults: Initially one 0.05 to 0.1 mg/d patch twice a week applied to the trunk (avoid breasts and waistline). Rotate application sites.

Contraindications: Undiagnosed abnormal genital bleeding; thromboembolic disorders; breast or estrogen-dependent carcinoma.

Precautions: History of breast cancer; cardiovascular disease; hepatic, renal, or cardiac insufficiency; asthma; epilepsy; migraine; endometriosis; depression; gallbladder disease; diabetes. Discontinue if hypertension or jaundice occurs and during immobilization or at least 4 weeks before surgery associated with increased risk of thromboembolism.

Adverse reactions: Increased risk of endometrial cancer or hyperplasia (add progesterone), thromboembolic disorders, increase in uterine fibromyomata size. Breakthrough bleeding; mastodynia; nausea; abdominal cramps; headache; migraine; dizziness; fluid retention; intolerance to contact lenses.

How supplied: Patch 0.05, 0.1, 0.2 mg/d

NOTES

ESTRATEST/ESTRATEST H.S.

ESTERIFIED ESTROGENS, METHYLTESTOSTERONE

Drug classes: Hormone/estrogen and testosterone

Pregnancy Category X

Indications:
- Moderate to severe menopausal vasomotor symptoms not improved by estrogens alone.
- Decreased libido

Adults: One tablet orally every day given with progesterone every day if patient has uterus, or cyclically (3 weeks on, 1 week off) with a progesterone D day 14-25 of cycle if patient is still having periods.

Contraindications: Breast or estrogen-dependent carcinoma; undiagnosed abnormal genital bleeding; thrombophlebitis; thromboembolic disorders or history of associated disorders with previous estrogen use; hepatic dysfunction.

Precautions: Cardiovascular disease; asthma; migraine; epilepsy; diabetes; renal dysfunction; gallbladder disease; bone disease associated with hypercalcemia; depression; uterine leiomyomas; discontinue if jaundice or hypertension occur.

Interactions: May potentiate oral anticoagulants and insulin.

Adverse reactions: Nausea; breakthrough bleeding; weight changes; mastalgia; hypertension; depression; hair loss or hirsutism; changes in libido; virilization; polycythemia; increased risk of endometrial carcinoma; gallbladder disease; thromboembolic disorders; hepatic tumors.

How supplied: Estratest: Tablet 1.25 mg estrogen with 2.5 mg methyltestosterone

Estratest H.S.: Tablet 0.625 mg with 1.25 mg methyltestosterone

NOTES

ETHAMBUTOL

MYAMBUTOL

Drug class: Antitubercular
Pregnancy Category B
Indications:

- Susceptible pulmonary tuberculosis

Adults: Give in one daily dose. Initially 15 mg orally/kg/day. Retreatment: 25 mg/kg/day. After 60 days, decrease dose to 15 mg/kg/day.
Contraindications: Optic neuritis; impaired renal function
Precautions: Use with other antituberculars. Test visual acuity before beginning therapy and periodically; monthly if dose exceeds 15 mg/kg/day.
Adverse reactions: Anaphylaxis; reduced visual acuity; optic neuritis; dermatitis; pruritus; joint pain; gastrointestinal upset; fever; malaise; headache; dizziness; confusion; peripheral neuritis; gout.
How supplied: Tablets 100, 400 mg

FAMVIR

FAMCICLOVIR SODIUM

Drug class: Antiviral
Pregnancy Category C
Indications:

- Management of acute herpes

Adults: Cold sores and genital lesions: 125 mg twice a day orally for 5 days. Shingles (herpes zoster): 500 mg every 8 hours orally for 7 days.
Contraindications: Contraindicated in presence of hypersensitivity to famciclovir or acyclovir. Use caution in the presence of cytopenia, impaired renal function.
  Use extreme caution with cytotoxic drugs because accumulation effect could cause severe bone marrow depression and other gastrointestinal and dermatologic problems. Lactation.
Adverse reactions: Headaches; diarrhea; fever; rash; cancer; and sterility.
How supplied: Tablets 125, 500 mg

FEMSTAT

BUTOCONAZOLE NITRATE

Drug class: Antifungal

Pregnancy Category C

Indications:

- Local treatment of vulvovaginal candidiasis

Adults: Pregnant patients: 1 applicator intravaginally at bedtime for 6 days. Nonpregnant patients: 1 applicator intravaginally at bedtime for 3 days.

Contraindications: Allergy to butoconazole or components used in preparation

Adverse reactions: Local—vulvovaginal burning, vulvar itching; discharge; soreness; swelling; itchy fingers

How supplied: Cream

FERROUS SULFATE

FEOSOL, FER-IRON, FEROSPACE, FERO-FOLIC-500

Drug class: Iron

Pregnancy Category A

Indications:

- Iron supplement

Adults: One to three tablets orally daily. Pregnancy: 325 to 600 mg orally daily in divided doses.

Contraindications: Hemochromatosis; gastrointestinal disease

Precautions: Hepatitis, pancreatitis, peptic ulcer. Monitor hemoglobin, hematocrit, reticulocyte.

Interactions: Inhibits tetracycline absorption. Best absorbed when taken between meals.

Adverse reactions: Nausea, abdominal discomfort, constipation, masks occult bleeding, black stools.

How supplied: Fero-folic-500 tablets: 525 mg ferrous sulfate plus 500 mg ascorbic acid and 1 mg folic acid; controlled release. **Fumarate tablets:** 63, 195, 200, 325 mg; controlled release: 300 mg. **Gluconate tablets:** 300, 350 mg; elixir: 300 mg/5 ml. **Sulfate tablets:** 300, 325 mg; extended-release capsules: 525 mg.

Fioricet

BUTALBITAL, ACETAMINOPHEN, CAFFEINE

Drug classes: Barbiturate, analgesic
Pregnancy Category C

Indications:
- Tension headache

Adults: One to two tablets every 4 hours; maximum: six daily
Contraindications: Allergy to ingredients
Precautions: Drug abusers; impaired hepatic or renal function; mental depression; suicidal tendencies; lactation
Adverse reactions: Drowsiness; dizziness; paradoxical excitement; gastrointestinal disturbances; mental depression; hepatotoxicity
How supplied: Tablets

Fiorinal

BUTALBITAL, ASPIRIN, CAFFEINE

Drug classes: Barbiturate, salicylate
Pregnancy Category C

Indications:
- Tension headache

Adults: One to two tablets every 4 hours; maximum: six daily
Contraindications: Nonsteroidal anti-inflammatory drug allergy; varicella or influenza in teenagers; porphyria; severe bleeding or coagulation disorders; peptic ulcer; gastritis; pregnancy; lactation.
Precautions: Drug abusers; asthma; impaired hepatic or renal function; gastritis. Monitor blood pressure, blood urea nitrogen, uric acid levels.
Adverse reactions: Drowsiness; dizziness; allergic reactions; paradoxical excitement; gastrointestinal disturbances; respiratory depression; salicylism.
How supplied: Tablets

Flagyl

METRONIDAZOLE

Drug class: Antiprotozoal

Pregnancy Category B

Indications:
- Bacterial vaginosis
- Trichomoniasis
- Pelvic inflammatory disease

Adults: Trichomoniasis: 250 mg orally three times a day for 1 week or 500 mg orally twice a day for 5 days. If not pregnant, 2 g orally at one time or 1 g AM, 1 g PM (divided dose) on same day. Pelvic inflammatory disease: 500 mg orally twice a day for 7 to 10 days.
  Also: Flagyl capsules: 375 mg orally twice a day for 5 days

Contraindications: First trimester of pregnancy.

Interactions: Avoid alcohol during and for 3 days after use. May potentiate oral anticoagulants, Phenytoin, Lithium. Antagonized by Phenobarbital, Phenytoin, other hepatic enzyme inducers.

Adverse reactions: Seizures; peripheral neuropathy; gastrointestinal upset; anorexia; constipation; headache; metallic taste; Candida overgrowth.

How supplied: Tablets 250, 375, 500 mg

Fleet Enema

SODIUM BIPHOSPHATE

Drug class: Laxative

Pregnancy Category C

Indications:
- Relief of constipation and bowel evacuant

Contraindications: Magacolon; signs/symptoms of appendicitis; congestive heart failure

Interactions: Electrolyte imbalances with calcium channel blockers. DO NOT use with diuretics.

Adverse reactions: Excessive bowel activity, perianal irritation, abdominal cramps

How supplied: Enema 59, 118 ml

FLOXIN

OFLOXACIN

Drug class: Antibacterial

Pregnancy Category C

Indications:

- Susceptible infections including genitourinary tract, cystitis

Adults: Oral: Take on empty stomach with full glass water; 200 to 400 mg every 12 hours for 7 days.

Contraindications: Contraindicated in the presence of allergy to fluoroquinolones.

Use caution in the presence of renal dysfunction; seizures; lactation.

Adverse reactions: Headache, dizziness, insomnia, nausea, fever, rash.

How supplied: Tablets 200, 300, 400 mg

FOLIC ACID

Drug class: Folic acid

Pregnancy Category A

Indications:

- Treatment of megaloblastic anemias due to sprue, nutritional deficiency, and pregnancy
- Prevention of neural tube defects in the fetus

Adults: Therapeutic dose: 400 to 800 µg/d orally. Prevention of neural tube defects: 1 to 2 mg/d orally. Start 3 to 4 months before pregnancy.

Contraindications: Contraindicated in the presence of allergies to folic acid preparations; pernicious, aplastic, normocytic anemias.

Precautions: Therapy may mask the signs of pernicious anemia.

Adverse reactions: Hypersensitivity; allergic reactions

How supplied: Tablets 0.1, 0.4, 1 mg

Fosamax

ALENDRONATE

Drug class: Aminobisphosphonate

Pregnancy Category C

Indications:

- Postmenopausal osteoporosis. Can increase bone density by up to 7% per year.

Adults: Take in the morning with a full glass of plain water at least 30 minutes before any other beverage, food, or medication; avoid recumbency for at least 30 minutes afterward. Postmenopausal osteoporosis: 10 mg/day; reevaluate periodically.

Contraindications: Hypocalcemia

Precautions: Upper gastrointestinal disease; renal dysfunction and lactation: not recommended. Assure adequate intake of vitamin D and calcium.

Interactions: Decreased absorption probable with food, calcium, and iron.

Adverse reactions: Gastrointestinal upset, musculoskeletal pain, headache.

How supplied: Tablets 10, 40 mg

Glycerin Suppository

GLYCEROL

Drug classes: Osmotic diuretic, hyperosmolar laxative

Pregnancy Category C

Indications:

- Constipation

Adults: Insert one suppository high in rectum and retain 15 minutes.

Contraindications: Hypersensitive to glycerin

Adverse reactions: Central nervous system: confusion, headache, syncope; gastrointestinal: nausea, vomiting

How supplied: Suppository

Hemabate

CARBOPROST TROMETHAMINE

Drug class: Prostaglandin
Pregnancy Category C

Indications:
- Postpartum hemorrhage due to uterine atony, which has not responded to conventional methods.

Adults: Refractory postpartum uterine bleeding: 250 µg intramuscular. May repeat in 5 to 15 minutes two times.
Contraindications: Allergy to prostaglandin preparations; active cardiac, hepatic, pulmonary, renal disease
Adverse reactions: Hypotension, nausea, flushing, dyspnea
How supplied: Intramuscular 250 µg in single dose vial

Hepatitis B Vaccine

ENGERIX-B, HEPTOVAX

Drug class: Hepatitis B vaccine
Pregnancy Category C

Indications:
- Hepatitis B Immunization

Adults: 20 µg intramuscular in deltoid muscle. Repeat 1 and 6 months later.
Contraindications: Yeast hypersensitivity
Precautions: Have epinephrine injection available. Pregnancy, lactation.
Adverse reactions: Local reactions, malaise, nausea, diarrhea, rash. Anaphylaxis.
How supplied: Injection: 10 mg/0.5 ml; 20 µg/ml

HYDROXYCHLOROQUINE

PLAQUENIL

Drug classes: Antimalarial, antirheumatic agent, 4-aminoquinoline

Pregnancy Category C

Indications:
- Malaria, amebiasis, and protozoal infections
- Chromic or acute rheumatoid arthritis
- Chronic discoid and systemic lupus erythematosus

Adults: 200 mg hydroxychloroquine sulfate equals 155 mg hydroxychloroquine base.
    Rheumatoid arthritis: Initial dose 400 to 600 mg/day orally taken with meals or milk. From 5 to 10 days later, gradually increase dosage to optimum effectiveness. Lupus erythematosus: 400 mg daily twice a day orally continued for several weeks or months; for prolonged use, 200 to 400 mg/day may be sufficient.

Contraindications: Allergy to 4-aminoquinolones, porphyria, psoriasis, retinal disease, and pregnancy. Caution with hepatic disease, alcoholism, G6PD deficiency.

Adverse reactions: Nausea, vomiting, diarrhea, blood dyscrasias, retinal and corneal changes, pruritus, bleaching of hair.

How supplied: Tablets 200 mg

IBUPROFEN

ADVIL, EXCEDRIN IB, IBUPRIN, MIDOL IB, MOTRIN, NUPRIN, PAMPRIN-IB

Drug classes: Nonsteroidal anti-inflammatory drug and nonnarcotic analgesic

Pregnancy Category B

Indications:
- Mild to moderate pain

Adults: 200 to 400 mg every 4 to 6 hours; maximum: 1.2 g/day

Contraindications: Aspirin allergy; pregnancy

Precautions: Gastrointestinal disease, impaired renal or hepatic function, lactation

Interactions: Avoid aspirin. May increase bleeding with anticoagulants, toxicity with methotrexate. Increases serum lithium levels.

Adverse reactions: Gastrointestinal problems, vision disorders, dizziness, rash, jaundice, hepatitis.

How supplied: Capsules 200, 400, 600, 800 mg

IMMUNE GLOBULIN (IG)

GAMASTAN, GAMMAR

Drug class: Biologicals

Pregnancy Category C

Indications:

- Prophylaxis after exposure to hepatitis A, rubeola, varicella, rubella—intramuscular preferable

Adults: Hepatitis A: 0.02 ml/kg, intramuscular; if traveling to areas where hepatitis A is common and staying less than 2 months, 0.06 ml/kg intramuscular repeated every 5 months for prolonged stay.

Rubeola: 0.2 ml/kg intramuscular if exposed less than 6 days previously. Varicella: 0.6 to 1.2 ml/kg intramuscular given promptly if zoster immune globulin unavailable. Rubella: 0.55 ml/kg intramuscular given to pregnant women exposed to rubella who will not consider abortion; may decrease likelihood of infection and fetal damage.

Contraindications: Allergy to gamma globulin or anti-immunoglobulin A antibodies

Use with caution on pregnant women—safety unestablished.

Adverse reactions: Tenderness; muscle stiffness at injection site; urticaria; angioedema; nausea; vomiting; chills; fever; chest tightness; anaphylactic reactions; abrupt fall in blood pressure—more likely with intravenous administration.

How supplied: Intravenous, intramuscular

NOTES

ISONIAZID

INH

Drug class: Antitubercular

Pregnancy Category C

Indications:

- Prophylaxis and treatment of susceptible tuberculosis

Adults: Prophylaxis: 300 mg orally daily. Active: 5 mg/kg daily; maximum: 300 mg every day; multiple drug therapy may be necessary.

Contraindications: Previous Isoniazid-associated hepatic injury; acute hepatic disease

Precautions: Impaired renal or hepatic function; diabetes; increased risk of liver damage with increasing age. Give concomitant Pyridoxine to decrease risk of neuropathy.

Interactions: Alcohol increases risk of hepatitis.

Adverse reactions: Hepatitis; peripheral neuropathy; gastrointestinal distress; blood dyscrasias; Pyridoxine deficiency; hyperglycemia; rheumatic and systemic lupus erythematosus-like syndrome.

How supplied: Tablets 300 mg

KEFLEX

CEPHALEXIN

Drug classes: Antibiotic and first generation cephalosporin

Pregnancy Category B

Indications:

- Susceptible infections including otitis media, skin, bone, respiratory or genitourinary tract

Adults: 250 to 500 mg orally every 6 hours for 5 to 7 days

Contraindications: Allergy to cephalosporins or penicillins; renal failure

Precautions: Impaired liver function; epilepsy; asthma; migraine; depression; cardiac or renal insufficiency

Adverse reactions: Anaphylaxis; diarrhea; rash; gastrointestinal upset; blood dyscrasias

How supplied: Capsules/tablets 250, 500 mg

MACROBID

NITROFURANTOIN

Drug class: Antibiotic
Pregnancy Category B
Indications:
- Susceptible urinary tract infections

Adults: 100 mg every 12 hours with meals for 7 days
Contraindications: Oliguria; pregnancy at term; lactation
Adverse reactions: Hemolytic anemia; nausea; headache; flatulence; dizziness; gastrointestinal disturbances; anorexia.
How supplied: Capsules 100 mg

MACRODANTIN

NITROFURANTOIN MACROCRYSTALS

Drug class: Antibiotic
Pregnancy Category B
Indications:
- Susceptible urinary tract infections

Adults: Take with food, 50 to 100 mg twice a day or four times a day for at least 7 days. Long-term suppressive use: 50 to 100 mg at bedtime.
Contraindications: Oliguria, lactation
Adverse reactions: Nausea; headache; flatulence; dizziness; gastrointestinal disturbances; anorexia; anaphylaxis
How supplied: Capsules: 25, 50, 100 mg

MAGNESIUM SULFATE

Drug classes: Electrolyte, anticonvulsant

Pregnancy Category A

Indications:
- Inhibition of premature labor
- Treatment of toxemia/eclampsia

Adults: Loading dose 4 g/250 ml in dextrose 5% in sterile H_2O (D_5W) intravenous in 15 minutes. Follow with 1 to 4 g every hour, not to exceed 3 ml/min.

Contraindications: Allergy to magnesium products; heart block; myocardial damage; abdominal pain, nausea, vomiting or other symptoms of appendicitis. Risk of magnesium toxicity in neonate if used in labor and delivery.

Interactions: Potentiation of neuromuscular blockade produced by nondepolarizing neuromuscular relaxants

Precautions: Administer only after calcium gluconate is available for magnesium toxicity.

Adverse reactions: Magnesium intoxication. Do magnesium level 2 to 4 hours after initiating treatment and every 4 to 6 hours as necessary. Hypocalcemia with tetany. Fetal depression.

How supplied: Injection, intravenous, intramuscular 10%, 50% sol; premixed bag 40 g in 1000 cc

METAMUCIL

PSYLLIUM

Drug class: Laxative (bulk)

Pregnancy Category C

Indications:
- Constipation

Adults: Dilute 1 tablespoon in 8 ounces of water or juice and take same time each day (preferably morning) for 2 to 3 days.

Contraindications: Allergy to bulk-forming laxatives. Symptoms of appendicitis, inflamed bowel or intestinal blockage.

Adverse reactions: Excessive bowel activity, abdominal cramps, cathartic dependence.

How supplied: Bulk, wafers

METHERGINE

METHYLERGONOVINE MALEATE

Drug class: oxytocic

Pregnancy Category C

Indications:
- Postpartum hemorrhage, uterine atony, subinvolution

Adults: 0.2 mg orally every 6 hours for six doses (maximum 1 week). 0.2 mg intramuscular every 2 to 4 hours after delivery as needed.

Contraindications: Hypertension

Interactions: Potentiated by vasoconstrictors, other ergot alkaloids

Adverse reactions: Hypertension or hypotension; stroke; nausea; vomiting; chest pain; dyspnea; dizziness; headache; hematuria; diarrhea; diaphoresis; palpitations.

How supplied: 0.2-mg tablets; 0.2-mg/ml ampules for injection

METROGEL-VAGINAL

METRONIDAZOLE 0.75%

Drug class: Vaginal antibiotic

Pregnancy Category B

Indications:
- Bacterial vaginosis

Adults: One full applicator vaginally twice daily for 5 days or 1 at bedtime for 5 to 7 days

Contraindications: Allergic to medication

Interactions: May potentiate oral anticoagulants

Adverse reactions: Local irritation, abdominal pain, nausea, dizziness

How supplied: Gel

MICRONOR

NORETHINDRONE

Drug class: Contraceptive

Pregnancy Category X

Indications:

- Oral contraception—preferred for nursing mothers because there is less affect on amount of milk production when compared to combination birth control pills.

Adults: Continuous regimen: 1 tablet orally daily without interruption. Start 6-week postpartum.

Contraindications: Thrombophlebitis or thromboembolic disorders; cerebrovascular or cardiovascular disease; undiagnosed abnormal genital bleeding.

Interactions: Antagonized by hepatic enzyme-inducing drugs, including anticonvulsants. Antacids and antibiotics may inhibit absorption.

Adverse reactions: Hypertension; nausea; vomiting; cramps; breakthrough bleeding; menstrual irregularities; changes in weight; mental depression; headache. (Contains no estrogen.)

How supplied: 28-day pack of 0.35-mg tablets

MILK OF MAGNESIA

MAGNESIUM HYDROXIDE

Drug classes: Laxative, Antacid

Pregnancy Category C

Indications:

- Upset stomach due to hyperacidity
- Hyperacidity due to peptic ulcer, gastritis, peptic esophagitis, gastric hyperacidity, hiatal hernia
- Prophylaxis of gastrointestinal bleeding, stress ulcers, aspiration pneumonia
- Constipation

Adults: Antacid: 5- to 15-ml liquid or 650-mg–to–1.3-g tablets orally four times a day. Laxative: 15 to 60 ml orally taken with liquid.

Contraindications: Allergy to magnesium products; caution in the presence of renal insufficiency

Adverse reactions: Diarrhea, nausea, perianal irritation

How supplied: Tablet or liquid

MONISTAT 7/MONISTAT 3

MICONAZOLE

Drug class: Vaginal infections
Pregnancy Category B

Indications:
- Vulvovaginal candidiasis
- Fungal skin infections

Adults: Vaginal Monostat 7: One applicator cream at bedtime for 7 days. Vaginal Monostat 3: 1 suppository vaginally daily at bedtime for 3 consecutive days. Cream to affected areas twice a day. If P_x for skin infection, continue treatment for 5 to 7 days after sores healed.

External: Apply cream to affected area twice a day.

Contraindications: Contraindicated in the presence of allergy to miconazole.

Adverse reactions: Allergic reactions with local swelling, and increased discharge.

How supplied: Vaginal suppository 100, 200 mg cream 2%. Monostat 3 combination pack of suppositories plus 0.32 oz of external vulvar cream

NIZORAL

KETOCONAZOLE 2%

Drug class: Antifungal
Pregnancy Category C

Indications:
- Tinea corporis, cruris, cutaneous, candidiasis, seborrheic dermatitis

Adults: Tablets: 200 mg orally every day for 3 weeks to 6 months depending on site, need for suppression. Cream: Apply once daily to affected and adjacent area. Treat for at least 2 weeks.

Seborrheic dermatitis: Apply to affected area twice daily for 4 weeks or until clinical clearing.

Contraindications: Hypersensitivity to the active or excipient ingredients of this formulation.

Adverse reactions: Tablets: Nausea, vomiting, headache, rash, thrombocytopenia; cream: severe irritation, pruritus, stinging, allergic reaction

How supplied: Tablets: 200 mg; cream; shampoo

NONOXYNOL 9

SEMICID

Drug class: Contraceptive spermicide

Pregnancy Category X

Indications:

- Contraception

Adults: One suppository vaginally at least 15 minutes and up to 1 hour before intercourse

Contraindications: Discontinue if irritation occurs.

How supplied: Suppository, VIF Film, coating in some condoms

NORPLANT

LEVONORGESTREL

Drug classes: Contraceptives, Progestin

Pregnancy Category X

Indications:

- Long-term (up to 5 years) contraception

Adults: Implant six Silastic capsules subdermally during the first 7 days of the onset of menses.

Contraindications: Active thrombophlebitis or thromboembolic disorders; undiagnosed abnormal genital bleeding; acute liver disease; benign or malignant liver tumors; breast cancer.

Interactions: Phenytoin and carbamazepine decrease efficacy of system

Adverse reactions: Local reactions or infection at insertion site; irregular menses; headache; nervousness; nausea; dizziness; mastalgia; weight gain; leukorrhea.

How supplied: One kit contains sterile supplies, six capsules each containing 36 mg levonorgestrel.

NUCOFED

Drug classes: Antitussive plus sympathomimetic
Pregnancy Category C

Indications:
- Nonproductive cough and congestion

Adults: One capsule every 6 hours as needed for cough. Nucofed expectorant: 5 ml every 6 hours as needed for cough.

Contraindications: Within 14 days of monoamine oxidase inhibitors; severe hypertension or cardiovascular disease; asthma; lower respiratory disorders

Adverse reactions: Central nervous system overstimulation; palpitations; headache; insomnia; drowsiness; convulsions; respiratory depression; urinary retention; constipation.

How supplied: Capsules, expectorant syrup

NYSTATIN 200,000 UNITS

MYCOSTATIN

Drug classes: Antifungal, antibiotic
Pregnancy category A

Indications:
- Treatment of oral candidiasis

Adults: 500,000 to 1,000,000 units three times a day. Continue for at least 48 hours after clinical cure.

Contraindications: Allergy to nystatin or components used in preparation

Adverse reactions: Diarrhea, gastrointestinal distress, nausea, vomiting, oral irritation

How supplied: Suspension: 60 ml (with dropper), 16 oz

OGEN 0.625 MG TABLETS/OGEN VAGINAL CREAM

ESTROPIPATE

Drug class: Estrogen
Pregnancy Category X

Indications:
- Hormone replacement therapy
- Atrophic vaginitis and moderate to severe vasomotor symptoms of menopause
- Osteoporosis prevention

Adults: Tablets: Menopause—0.625 to 1.25 mg orally daily, or cycle 3 weeks on and 1 week off; cream: 2 to 4 g vaginally daily; give daily at bedtime for 1 week, every other day for 1 week, maintenance dose one to two times per week

Contraindications: Breast or estrogen-dependent carcinoma; undiagnosed abnormal genital bleeding; thromboembolic disorders; thrombophlebitis

Precautions: Cardiovascular disease; asthma; migraine; epilepsy; hepatic or renal dysfunction; gallbladder disease; uterine leiomyomas. Discontinue if jaundice or hypertension occur and during immobilization or at least 4 weeks before surgery.

Adverse reactions: Nausea; vomiting; breakthrough bleeding; weight changes; swollen and tender breasts; hypertension; mental depression; increased size of uterine fibroma. Increased risk of estrogen-dependent carcinoma if given without progesterone in a woman with a uterus; gallbladder disease; thromboembolic disorders; hepatic tumors.

How supplied: Tablets 0.625, 1.25 mg; cream

PHENERGAN/PHENERGAN VC

Drug classes: Antipertussis, Phenergan VC: Narcotic
Pregnancy Category C

Indications:
- Cough
- Nasal congestion
- Symptoms associated with the common cold

Adults: One teaspoon orally every 4 to 6 hours as necessary

Contraindications: Diabetes, peptic ulcer, pregnancy, lactation, and allergy to ingredients

Caution: With history of alcohol or drug dependence

Adverse reactions: Drowsiness, dizziness

How supplied: Liquid Phenergan: 0.625 mg Promethazine plus 15 mg Dextromethorpan; liquid Phenergan VC: 0.625 mg Promethazine plus 15 mg Dextromethorpan plus 10 mg codeine

PITOCIN

OXYTOCIN

Drug classes: Oxytocic, hormonal agent

Pregnancy Category C

Indications:

- Antepartum to initiate or improve uterine contractions
- Postpartum to produce uterine contractions during the third stage of labor and to control postpartum bleeding

Adults: Induction or stimulation of labor: Initial dose of no more than 1 to 2 mU/min (0.001 to 0.002 U/min) by intravenous infusion through an infusion pump. Increase dose in increments of no more than 1 to 2 mU/min at 15- to 30-minute intervals until a contraction pattern similar to normal labor is established. DO NOT exceed 20 mU/min. Discontinue in event of uterine hyperactivity, fetal distress. Control of postpartum uterine bleeding: intravenous drip—add 10 to 40 units to 1000 ml of a nonhydrating diluent, run at a rate to control uterine atony; intramuscular: administer 10 units after delivery of placenta.

Contraindications: Significant cephalopelvic disproportion; unfavorable fetal positions or presentation; hypertonic uterine patterns; induction or augmentation of labor when vaginal delivery is contraindicated

Adverse reactions: Nausea, vomiting, cardiac arrhythmias, postpartum hemorrhage, fetal bradycardia

How supplied: Ampules 10 units in 1 ml

NOTES

PREDNISOLONE

DELTA-CORTEF, NOVOPREDNISOLONE (CAN), PRELONE

Drug classes: Adrenal corticosteroid, hormonal agent

Pregnancy Category C

Indications:
- Short-term inflammatory allergic, dermatologic diseases, status asthmaticus, and autoimmune disorders (systemic)
- Hematologic disorders: thrombocytopenia purpura, erythroblastopenia (systemic)

Adults: Oral, intramuscular, or intravenous: 5 to 60 mg/day. Increase until lowest effective dose is reached. Decrease slowly if therapy is long term; DO NOT suddenly stop.

Contraindications: Contraindicated in presence of infections, especially tuberculosis; fungal infections; amebiasis; vaccinia and varicella and antibiotic-resistant infections; lactation. Caution with kidney or liver disease; hypothyroidism; active or latent peptic ulcer; inflammatory bowel disease; congestive heart failure; hypertension; thromboembolic disorders; osteoporosis; convulsive disorders; diabetes mellitus. Suppresses skin test reactions.

Adverse reactions: Vertigo; headache; increased appetite; weight gain with long-term therapy; sodium and fluid retention; immunosuppression; aggravation or masking of infections; impaired wound healing. Increased toxic effects of prednisolone if taken concurrently with estrogens (includes oral contraceptives). Decreased steroid blood levels when taken with barbiturates, phenytoin, rifampin. Decreased effectiveness of salicylates when taken with prednisolone.

How supplied: Tablets, liquid

NOTES

PREDNISONE

APO-PREDNISONE (CAN), DELTASONE, PANASOL

Drug classes: Adrenal corticosteroid, hormonal agent

Pregnancy Category C

Indications:

- Short-term inflammatory and allergic; dermatologic diseases; status asthmaticus; autoimmune disorders
- Hematologic disorders: thrombocytopenia purpura, erythroblastopenia

Adults: Depends on severity of condition and patient's response. Administer daily dose before 9 AM to minimize adrenal suppression. For long-term therapy, alternate therapy should be considered. After long-term therapy, withdrawal should be slow to avoid adrenal insufficiency. Initial dose: 30 mg/day orally; maintenance: reduce or increase in small 5-mg increments at intervals until satisfactory response is reached.

Contraindications: Contraindicated in presence of infections, especially tuberculosis; fungal infections; amebiasis; vaccinia and varicella and antibiotic resistant infections; lactation. Caution with kidney or liver disease; hypothyroidism; active or latent peptic ulcer; inflammatory bowel disease; congestive heart failure; hypertension; thromboembolic disorders; osteoporosis; convulsive disorders; diabetes mellitus. Suppresses skin test reactions.

Adverse reactions: Vertigo; headache; increased appetite; weight gain with long-term therapy; sodium and fluid retention; immunosuppression; aggravation or masking of infections; impaired wound healing. Increased toxic effects of prednisone if taken concurrently with estrogens (includes oral contraceptives). Decreased steroid blood levels when taken with barbiturates, phenytoin, rifampin. Decreased effectiveness of salicylates when taken with prednisone.

How supplied: Tablets 1, 2.5, 5, 10, 25, 50 mg

NOTES

PREMARIN (ORAL/CREAM)

CONJUGATED ESTROGENS

Drug class: Hormone, synthetic estrogen

Pregnancy Category X

Indications:
- Moderate to severe vasomotor symptoms associated with menopause
- Vaginal atrophy
- Osteoporosis prevention

Adults: Hormone replacement therapy: Usual dose 0.625 or 1.25 mg one orally every day. Maybe given days 1 to 25 of each menstrual cycle. **Must** be given with a progestin unless patient has a hysterectomy.

Atrophic vaginitis: One applicator vaginally daily at bedtime for 1 week then every other day for 1 week; decrease to two for week. Maintenance: one to two for 1 week

Contraindications: Breast or estrogen-dependent carcinoma; active thrombophlebitis or thromboembolic disorders; undiagnosed abnormal genital bleeding

Precautions: Asthma; epilepsy; migraine; diabetes; cardiac or renal dysfunction; depression. Discontinue if jaundice; visual disturbances; migraine; or thrombotic disorders occur.

Adverse reactions: Thromboembolic events; edema; cholestatic jaundice; depression; pyrexia; insomnia; nausea; breast tenderness; galactorrhea

How supplied: Tablets 0.3, 0.625, 0.9, 1.25, 2.5 mg; cream

NOTES

PREMPHASE

Drug classes: Estrogen and progestin

Pregnancy Category X

Indications:
- Moderate to severe vasomotor symptoms associated with menopause
- Vulvar and vaginal atrophy
- Osteoporosis prevention

Adults: One tablet orally of Premarin 0.625 mg every day. Tablets 15 to 28 contain 5 mg of Cycrin as well

Contraindications: Breast or estrogen-dependent carcinoma; active thrombophlebitis or thromboembolic disorders; undiagnosed abnormal genital bleeding; hepatic impairment

Precautions: Gallbladder disease; monitor blood pressure; discontinue if visual abnormalities occur; asthma; migraine; epilepsy; cardiac or renal dysfunction

Adverse reactions: Nausea; vomiting; cramps; swelling or tenderness of the abdomen; hepatic impairment; breast tenderness or enlargement; uterine fibroids; breakthrough bleeding or spotting; headache; migraine; dizziness; changes in vision; depression; glucose intolerance

How supplied: First blister card: 14 tablets of Premarin 0.625 mg; second blister card: 14 tablets of Premarin 0.625 mg plus Cycrin 5 mg

NOTES

PREMPRO

Drug classes: Estrogen and progestin
Pregnancy Category X

Indications:
- Moderate to severe vasomotor symptoms associated with menopause
- Osteoporosis prevention

Adults: Take one tablet containing Premarin and Cycrin daily.

Contraindications: Breast or estrogen-dependent carcinoma; active thrombophlebitis or thromboembolic disorders; undiagnosed abnormal genital bleeding; hepatic impairment

Precautions: Gallbladder disease; monitor blood pressure; hypercalcemia in breast cancer. Discontinue if visual abnormalities occur. Asthma, migraine, epilepsy, cardiac or renal dysfunction.

Adverse reactions: Nausea; vomiting; cramps; swelling or tenderness of the abdomen; hepatic impairment; breast tenderness or enlargement; uterine fibroids; breakthrough bleeding or spotting; headache; migraine; dizziness; changes in vision; depression; glucose intolerance

How supplied: Two blister cards—28 tablets of Premarin 0.625 mg and Cycrin 2.5 mg

PREPARATION H

Drug class: Live yeast cell derivative

Indications:
- Hemorrhoids

Adults: Apply freely externally three to five times daily. Suppository: One rectally in AM and PM and after each evacuation.

Adverse reactions: Discontinue if local irritation occurs—redness, pain, swelling.

How supplied: Ointment, cream, suppository

PROBENECID

BENEMID

Drug classes: Uricosuric, sulfonamide derivative
Pregnancy Category B

Indications:

- Adjunct in penicillin/cephalosporin treatment

Adults: One g orally with 3.5 g ampicillin or 1 g 30 minutes before before 4 to 8 million units of aqueous penicillin G procaine intramuscular

Contraindications: Hypersensitivity, hepatic disease, severe renal disease

Interactions: Increased activity oral anticoagulants; increased toxicity sulfa drugs; Para-aminosalicyclic acid (PAS), rifampin, naproxen

Adverse reactions: Headache, drowsiness, bradycardia, glycosuria, and thirst

How supplied: Tablets 0.5 g

PROCTOFOAM-HC

Drug classes: Antipruritic and steroid
Pregnancy Category C

Indications:

- Steroid responsive anogenital dermatoses

Adults: Apply three to four times daily

Precautions: Tuberculosis; diverticulitis; treat infection if present. Significant systemic absorption may occur. Discontinue if no improvement in 2 to 3 weeks. Lactation.

Adverse reactions: Adrenal suppression; dermal and epidermal atrophy; poor wound healing; local irritation; folliculitis; hypertrichosis; hypopigmentation; macerations; secondary infections; striae; miliaria

How supplied: Aerosol, cream

PROGESTERONE IN OIL

Drug class: Hormone progestin

Pregnancy Category X

Indications:
- Treatment of secondary amenorrhea

Adults: Amenorrhea: 100 mg intramuscular. Expect withdrawal bleeding 48 to 72 hours. Spontaneous normal cycles may follow.

Contraindications: Allergy to progestins; thromboembolic disorders; cerebral hemorrhage or history of these conditions; hepatic disease; missed abortion. Use caution in the presence of epilepsy; migraine; asthma; cardiac or renal dysfunction.

Adverse reactions: Dizziness; thrombophlebitis; breakthrough bleeding; spotting; change in menstrual flow

How supplied: Injection intramuscular 25, 50, 100 mg/ml

PROMETHAZINE HCL

PHENERGAN SUPPOSITORY, INTRAMUSCULAR

Drug classes: Antiemetic

Pregnancy Category C

Indications:
- Nausea and vomiting
- Motion sickness

Adults: Orally: 25 mg every 4 to 6 hours as necessary; intramuscular: 12.5 to 25 mg every 4 hours as necessary

Suppository: 25 mg rectally, repeat in 4 to 6 hours, as needed. Motion sickness: 25 mg orally twice a day

Contraindications: Hypersensitivity to antihistamines or phenothiazines

Interactions: Potentiates central nervous system depression with alcohol and other central nervous system depressants. May alter human chorionic gonadotropin pregnancy test results.

Adverse reactions: Drowsiness; lowered seizure threshold; cholestatic jaundice; rash

How supplied: Tablets: 12.5, 25, 50 mg; intramuscular: 25, 50 mg/ml

PROSTIN E2, PREPIDIL GEL

DINOPROSTONE

Drug class: Prostaglandin
Pregnancy Category C

Indications:
- Induction of labor, initiation of cervical ripening

Adults: Insert one Prostin E2 dose into cervical os every 2 hours three times. Prepidil: One dose into cervical os. Repeat 6 hours later as necessary.

Contraindications: Allergy to prostaglandin preparations; active cardiac; hepatic; pulmonary; renal disease. Malposition of fetus, hypertonic contractions; fetal distress.

Adverse reactions: Drowsiness; confusion; nervousness; epigastric distress; nausea; vomiting; diarrhea; hypotension; palpitations; tachycardia

How supplied: PGE2: suppository 20 mg

PGE2 and Prepidil gel: premixed single dose in syringe with insertion catheter

PROVENTIL INHALER

ALBUTEROL

Drug class: $\beta 2$ agonist
Pregnancy Category C

Indications:
- Bronchospasm
- Asthma

Adults: One to two inhalations every 4 to 6 hours as needed. Exercise-induced bronchospasm: 2 inhalations 15 minutes before exercise

Contraindications: Hypersensitivity to albuterol; heart disease; hypertension

Adverse reactions: Tachycardia; hypertension; tremor; nervousness; headache; dizziness; hyperactivity; insomnia; nausea; muscle cramps; paradoxical bronchospasm; local irritation

How supplied: Inhalation: 17 g (200 inhalations)

PROVERA

MEDROXYPROGESTERONE ACETATE

Drug class: Progestogen

Pregnancy Category X

Indications:

- Secondary amenorrhea
- Abnormal uterine bleeding due to hormonal imbalance without organic pathology
- In hormone replacement therapy with estrogen to protect against endometrial cancer

Adults: Amenorrhea: 5 to 10 mg daily for 5 to 10 days. Cyclic hormone replacement therapy or abnormal bleeding: 5 to 10 mg daily for 10 to 12 days starting on days 14 to 16 of menstrual cycle or for the first 10 to 12 days of each month; to induce optimum secretory transformation or primed endometrium. Hormone replacement therapy: Continuous dose of 2.5 or 5 mg every day with an estrogen.

Contraindications: Active thrombophlebitis or thromboembolic disorders; cerebral apoplexy; hepatic dysfunction or disease; undiagnosed abnormal vaginal bleeding; pregnancy

Precautions: Asthma; epilepsy; migraine; diabetes; cardiac or renal dysfunction; depression

Adverse reactions: Thromboembolic events; edema; depression; insomnia; nausea; acne; hirsutism; alopecia; rash

How supplied: Tablets 2.5, 5, 10 mg

NOTES

PYRAZINAMIDE

PYRAZINAMIDE

Drug class: Nicotinamide analogue
Pregnancy Category C

Indications:
- Susceptible pulmonary tuberculosis

Adults: 15 to 30 mg/kg orally once daily; maximum: 2 g daily. Or 50 to 70 mg/kg twice weekly based on lean body weight
Contraindications: Severe hepatic damage; acute gout
Precautions: Use with other antituberculars. Monitor hepatic function and serum uric acid before and during therapy. Hepatocellular damage or hyperuricemia with acute gouty arthritis, discontinue. Diabetics may be harder to control. Lactation.
Interactions: May interfere with Acetest or Ketostix
Adverse reactions: Hepatitis; liver dysfunction; gout; gastrointestinal disturbances; arthralgia; myalgia; blood dyscrasias
How supplied: Tablets 500 mg

RHOGAM

RHO(D) IMMUNE GLOBULIN HUMAN

Drug class: Immunomodulators
Pregnancy Category C

Indications:
- Preventing Rho(D) sensitization in nonsensitized Rho(D)-negative or Du-negative patients to the Rho(D) factor, following pregnancy or accidental transfusion

Adults: Each vial or syringe prevents sensitization to a volume of up to 15 ml of Rh-positive packed red blood cells. Administer intramuscularly at 28 weeks of gestation, within 72 hours of an Rh incompatible delivery, miscarriage, abortion, or transfusion accident. Use MICRhoGAM for abortions less than 12 weeks.
Contraindications: Rho(D) positive patients
Adverse reactions: Local reactions
How supplied: Single-dose syringes; MICRhoGAM: single-dose syringes

RIFAMPIN

RIFADIN

Drug class: Rifamycin
Pregnancy Category C

Indications:
- Susceptible pulmonary tuberculosis

Adults: 600 mg orally daily. Give 1 hour before or 2 hours after meals.

Contraindications: Contraindicated in the presence of allergy to any rifamycin; acute hepatic disease. Use caution in pregnancy, lactation.

Interactions: Phenytoin and carbamazepine decrease efficacy of system.

Adverse reactions: Increases microsomal hepatic enzyme metabolism. Avoid use within 8 hours of PAS. Concomitant ketoconazole decreases serum concentration of both drugs.

How supplied: 150, 300 mg

ROCEPHIN

CEFTRIAXONE SODIUM

Drug classes: Antibiotic/cephalosporin
Pregnancy Category B

Indications:
- Susceptible bacterial septicemia
- Lower respiratory or urinary tract
- Skin and skin structure, bone and joint
- Gynecologic, intra-abdominal infections
- Meningitis
- Gonorrhea
- Surgical prophylaxis

Adults: 1 to 2 mg intramuscular or intravenous daily or in two equally divided doses; maximum: 4 g/day. Gonorrhea: One dose of 250 mg intramuscular.

Precautions: Penicillin or other allergy; concomitant renal and hepatic impairment

Interactions: Potentiated by probenecid

Adverse reactions: Anaphylaxis, elevated liver enzymes. Local reactions, rash, diarrhea, nausea, vomiting.

How supplied: Vials 250, 500 mg; 1, 2 g

RUBELLA VIRUS VACCINE

MERUVAX II

Drug class: Rubella virus live

Pregnancy Category C

Indications:

- Rubella immunization

Adults: 12 months and over: single subcutaneous injection

Contraindications: Hypersensitivity to neomycin. Active respiratory or other febrile infection. Active untreated tuberculosis. Immune deficiency. Pregnancy during and up to 3 months after vaccination.

Precautions: Have epinephrine injection available. Defer vaccination for at least 3 months after blood or plasma transfusions or immune serum globulin, and for at least 1 month before or after other live virus vaccines. Lactation.

Adverse reactions: Malaise; rash; fever; headache; local reactions; arthritic symptoms; thrombocytopenic purpura; encephalitis

How supplied: Single-dose vial

SENOKOT

DOCUSATE SODIUM/SENNA

Drug class: Laxative (emollient)

Pregnancy Category C

Indications:

- Constipation

Adults: One to eight tablets a day at bedtime

Contraindications: Allergy to emollient laxatives. Abdominal pain and fever related to appendicitis.

Adverse reactions: Abdominal cramping and discomfort

How supplied: Tablets

SLOW FE/SLOW FE PLUS FOLIC ACID

IRON

Drug class: Iron supplement
Pregnancy Category A

Indications:
- Prevention and treatment of iron deficiency anemias

Adults: One tablet daily
Contraindications: Hemochromatosis; hemosiderosis
Interactions: Inhibits tetracycline absorption
Adverse reactions: Nausea; abdominal discomfort and pain; constipation; diarrhea
How supplied: Time-release tablets; time-release tablets with folic acid

SPECTINOMYCIN

TROBICIN

Drug class: Antibiotic
Pregnancy category B

Indications:
- Gonorrhea

Adults: Two to four grams as single dose
Contraindications: Allergy to spectinomycin, lactation
Caution: Pregnancy (safety not established)
Adverse reactions: Dizziness; chills; decreased urine output without documented renal toxicity; soreness at injection site
How supplied: Intramuscular 2, 4 g

STADOL

BUTORPHANOL TARTRATE

Drug class: Opioid (partial agonist)

Pregnancy Category C

Indications:
- Pain management when opioid analgesia appropriate

Adults: Intramuscular: 1 to 4 mg every 3 to 4 hours; intravenous: 1 to 2 mg every 3 to 4 hours as needed

Precautions: Impaired respiratory, cardiac, renal or hepatic function; hypertension; drug abusers

Interactions: Potentiation with alcohol, central nervous system depressants. May precipitate withdrawal in narcotic addicts.

Adverse reactions: Sedation, dizziness, gastrointestinal upset; respiratory depression; diaphoresis; hypotension; hypertension; rash

How supplied: Injection (vials) 1, 2 mg/ml

SUDAFED/SUDAFED 12 HOUR CAPSULES

PSEUDOEPHEDRINE HCL

Drug class: Sympathomimetic

Pregnancy Category C

Indications:
- Nasal and eustachian tube congestion

Adults: Sudafed: One tablet orally every 4 to 6 hours; Sudafed 12 hour: One tablet orally every 12 hours

Contraindications: Severe hypertension or cardiovascular disease; during or within 14 days of monoamine oxidase inhibitors

Interactions: Hypertensive crisis with MAOIs. β-blockers increase pressor effects of sympathomimetics. Arrhythmias with epinephrine, isoproterenol. Antagonizes methyldopa, reserpine, guanethidine.

Adverse reactions: Central nervous system overstimulation; palpitations; headache; hypertension; dizziness; gastrointestinal disturbances; nervousness; tremor; weakness; pallor; dysuria; insomnia; convulsions

How supplied: Tablets: 30, 60, 120 mg; capsule extended release: 120 mg

TERAZOL 3/TERAZOL 7/TERAZOL CREAM

TERCONAZOLE

Drug class: Antifungal
Pregnancy Category C

Indications:
- Vulvovaginal candidiasis
- Fungal infections of the skin

Adults: Vaginal cream: One full applicator vaginally at bedtime for 3 or 7 consecutive nights; one suppository vaginally at bedtime for 3 consecutive nights. Skin: apply twice a day to affected area until all evidence of infection has been gone for 5 to 7 days.

Precautions: Confirm diagnosis by potassium hydroxide smears. Discontinue if fever, chills, irritation, or sensitization occurs.

Adverse reactions: Headache, fever, chills, itching, body pain (cream); localized burning, genital pain, and fever (suppository); dysmenorrhea (3 cream)

How supplied: Cream 3 day, 7 day; suppository: 3 day

TERBUTALINE

TERBUTALINE SULFATE

Drug class: Tocolytic
Pregnancy Category B

Indications:
- Inhibition of premature labor

Adults: Premature labor: Initiate intravenous administration at 10 µg/min. Titrate upward to a maximum of 80 µg/min. Maintain at minimum effective dosage for 4 hours. Oral doses of 2.5 to 5 mg orally every 4 to 6 hours have been used as maintenance therapy

Contraindications: Hypersensitivity to terbutaline; tachyarrhythmias; unstable vasomotor system disorders; hypertension

Interactions: Increased likelihood of cardiac arrhythmias when given with halogenated hydrocarbon anesthetics, cyclopropane

Adverse reactions: Restlessness; apprehension; anxiety; fear; nausea; cardiac arrhythmias; palpitations; respiratory difficulties; pulmonary edema

How supplied: Tablets: 2.5, 5 mg; ampules: 1 mg/ml

TETRACYCLINE

Drug classes: Antibiotic, tetracycline
Pregnancy Category B

Indications:
- Tetracycline-sensitive infections

Adults: Take 1 hour before or 2 hours after meals. 250 to 500 mg four times a day for 7 days.

Contraindications: Allergy to any of the tetracyclines; pregnancy; lactation. Use caution in the presence of hepatic or renal dysfunction.

Interactions: May increase digoxin levels. Food reduces absorption.

Adverse reactions: Superinfections; photosensitivity; gastrointestinal upset; enterocolitis; rash; blood dyscrasias; increased blood urea nitrogen; hepatotoxicity

How supplied: Tablets: 250, 500 mg

TIGAN

TRIMETHOBENZAMIDE HCL

Drug class: Antiemetic
Pregnancy Category C

Indications:
- Nausea and vomiting

Adults: Capsules: 250 mg three to four times daily; suppository: 200 mg rectally three to four times daily; injection: 200 mg intramuscular three to four times daily. Precautions: Pregnancy, lactation.

Interactions: Potentiates alcohol, other central nervous system depressants

Adverse reactions: Extrapyramidal reactions; may mask emetic signs of disease; drowsiness; blood dyscrasias; blurred vision; coma; seizures; depression; diarrhea; dizziness; jaundice; hypotension (injection); headache; muscle cramps; opisthotonos.

How supplied: Capsules 100, 200 mg; suppositories: 200 mg; ampules: 100 mg/ml

Tums

CALCIUM CARBONATE

Drug classes: Antacid, electrolyte

Pregnancy Category C

Indications:
- Hyperacidity in upper gastrointestinal tract, including stomach and esophagus; heartburn or acid indigestion
- Diseases include peptic ulcer, gastritis, esophagitis, hiatal hernia

Adults: Recommended daily allowance: 800 mg; 1200 mg pregnancy. Dietary supplement: 500 mg to 2 g orally, twice to four times a day. Antacid: .05 to 2.0 g orally

Contraindications: Allergy to calcium; renal calculi; hypercalcemia; patients with risk of existing digitalis toxicity. False negative values for serum and urinary magnesium.

Adverse reactions: Slowed heart rate, tingling, "heat waves" (rapid intravenous administered); peripheral vasodilation; local burning; anorexia; nausea; vomiting; constipation; rebound hyperacidity; local irritation. Decreased absorption of oral calcium when taken concurrently with oxalic acid (in rhubarb and spinach); phytic acid (bran and whole cereals); phosphorus (dairy products).

How supplied: Tablets or wafers

Tylenol

ACETAMINOPHEN

Drug class: Analgesic

Pregnancy Category B

Indications:
- Mild to moderate pain
- Fever

Adults: 325 to 650 mg every 4 to 6 hours

Contraindications: Allergy to acetaminophen. Use caution in the presence of impaired hepatic function, chronic alcoholism.

Adverse reactions: Rash; hepatotoxicity (overdosage)

How supplied: Tablets: 325 mg; gel tablets: 500 mg

TYLENOL NO. 3

ACETAMINOPHEN WITH CODEINE

Drug class: Analgesics
Pregnancy Category C

Indications:
- Mild to moderately severe pain

Adults: One to two tablets every 4 to 6 hours as necessary for pain

Precautions: Head injury; acute abdomen; impaired renal, hepatic, thyroid, or adrenocortical function; asthma; drug abusers; lactation

Interactions: Potentiation with alcohol; central nervous system depressants, monoamine oxidase inhibitors; tricyclic antidepressants; anticholinergics

Adverse reactions: Dizziness; sedation; nausea; vomiting; constipation; urinary retention; rash; respiratory depression; hepatotoxicity (overdosage)

How supplied: Tablet: No. 3—acetaminophen 300 mg with codeine phosphate 30 mg

UNISOM

DOXYLAMINE SUCCINATE

Drug classes: Antihistamine, mild sedative
Pregnancy Category C

Indications:
- Insomnia
- Nausea aid in pregnancy when used with B_6
- Hayfever, hives, rash, or itching

Adults: Insomnia: One to two tablets orally at bedtime; nausea: 1/2 Unisom tablet with 25 mg B_6 orally four times a day as necessary; hayfever: 25 mg orally four times a day

How supplied: Tablets: 25 mg

VISTARIL, ATARAX, ANXANIL

HYDROXYZINE HYDROCHLORIDE

Also: Atarax Syrup Hydroxyzine HCl 10 mg/5 ml; alcohol 0.5%
Drug classes: Antihistamine, antianxiety, antiemetic
Pregnancy Category C

Indications:
- Anxiety
- Management of pruritus due to allergic conditions
- Preoperatively/postoperatively

Adults: 25 to 100 mg orally twice to four times a day. 25 to 100 mg intramuscular every 4 to 6 hours
Contraindications: Early pregnancy
Precautions: Therapy for more than 4 months
Interactions: Potentiates central nervous system depression with alcohol and other central nervous system depressants
Adverse reactions: Drowsiness, dry mouth, tremor, convulsions
How supplied: Tablets: 10, 265, 50, 100, 500 mg; injection: 50 to 100 mg

ZANTAC

RANITIDINE

Drug class: Histamine antagonist
Pregnancy Category B

Indications:
- Active duodenal or benign gastric ulcer
- Gastroesophageal disease

Adults: 150 mg orally twice a day; 300 mg orally at bedtime.
Contraindications: Allergy to ranitidine
Interactions: Increased effects of warfarin; tricyclic antidepressants taken with rantidine. Decreased effectiveness of Diazepam if taken concurrently.
Adverse reactions: Headache; gastrointestinal disturbances; jaundice; hepatitis; rash; central nervous system disturbances; arrhythmias; arthralgia; myalgia; blood dyscrasias; anaphylaxis
How supplied: Tablets and capsules 150, 300 mg; intramuscular: 25 mg/ml

ZIDOVUDINE

See AZT (page 262).

ZITHROMAX

AZITHROMYCIN

Drug classes: Antibacterial, macrolide antibiotic

Pregnancy Category B

Indications:

- Mild to moderate susceptible infections including respiratory tract, uncomplicated skin and skin structures, nongonococcal urethritis, chlamydia, cervicitis

Adults: Take 1 hour before meals or 2 hours after. 500 mg day 1, then 250 mg daily for 4 days. Nongonococcal urethritis, chlamydia: 1 g as a single dose.

Oral suspension (zithromax cocktail): single-dose packet. Mix the entire contents of the packet with two ounces of water. Drink the entire contents immediately. Add an additional two ounces of water. Mix and drink all of that liquid. Can take with or without food.

Precautions: Renal or hepatic impairment; monitor for superinfection; hypersensitivity

Interactions: Avoid concomitant antacids

Adverse reactions: Gastrointestinal upset; abdominal pain; vaginitis; cholestatic jaundice

How supplied: Capsules: 250 mg; 2-pack (six capsules); oral suspension: one dose pack

Bibliography

Abramowicz M. *The Medical Letter.* 37th ed. New Rochelle, NY: The Medical Letter Inc; 1995:964.
Aikins Murphy P. Periconceptional supplementation with folic acid: Does it prevent neural tube defects? *J Nurse Midwifery.* 1992;37(1):25–32.
American Academy of Pediatrics, American College of Obstetricians and Gynecologists. *Guidelines for Perinatal Care.* 3rd ed. Elk Grove Village, IL: American Academy of Pediatrics; 1992.
American College of Nurse-Midwives. *Philosophy.* Washington, DC: Author, 1978.
American College of Obstetricians and Gynecologists. *Women's Health: The Menopause Years.* Washington, DC: Author, 1992.
American College of Obstetricians and Gynecologists. *ACOG Technical Bulletin—Management of Hypertension in Pregnancy.* Washington, DC: Author, 1994.
American Society of Hospital Pharmacists. Contraceptives estrogen-progestin combinations. *American Hospital Formulary Service Drug Information.* 1993; 68:1924–1929.
Andolina VF, Lille S, Willison KM. *Mammographic Imaging.* Philadelphia: JB Lippincott, 1992.
Apgar V. A proposal for a new method of evaluation of the newborn infant. *Current Research in Anesthesia and Analgesia.* 1953;32:260–267.
Baines C. Physical examination of the breasts in screening for breast cancer. *J Gerontol.* 1992;47:63–67.
Bargar M, Fullerton J, Lops V, Rhode MA, eds. *Protocols for Gynecologic and Obstetric Health Care.* Philadelphia: WB Saunders, 1988.
Butz AM, Hutton N, Joyner M, et al. HIV-infected women and infants: Social and health factors impeding utilization of health care. *J Nurse Midwifery.* 1993;38(2):103–109.
Byyny RL, Speroff L. *A Clinical Guide for the Care of Older Women.* Baltimore: Williams & Wilkins, 1990.
Cabaniss CD, Cabaniss ML. Physiologic hematology of pregnancy. In: Kitay DZ, ed. *Hematologic Problems in Pregnancy.* Oradell, NJ: Medical Economics Books, 1987.
CCS Publishing. *Current Clinical Strategies: Gynecology and Obstetrics.* Newport Beach, RI: Author, 1992.
Centers for Disease Control and Prevention. 1989 Sexually transmitted diseases treatment guidelines. *MMWR* 1989; 38 (Suppl. S-8).

Clark-Coller T. Dysfunctional uterine bleeding and amenorrhea: Differential diagnosis and management. *J Nurse Midwifery.* 1991;36(1): 49–62.

Cook MJ. Perimenopause: An opportunity for health promotion. *J Obst Gynecol Neonatal Nurs.* 1993;22(3):223–228.

Corbett JV. *Laboratory Tests and Diagnostic Procedures with Nursing Diagnosis.* Norwalk, CT: Appleton & Lange, 1992.

Crowell DT. Weight change in the postpartum period. *J Nurse Midwifery.* 1995;40:418–423.

Crum C, Newkirk G. Abnormal Pap smears, cancer risk, and HPV. *Patient Care.* 1995; :35–61.

Cunningham FG, MacDonald P, Grant N. *Williams Obstetrics.* 18th ed. Norwalk, CT: Appleton & Lange, 1989.

Cunningham FG, MacDonald P, Grant N, Leveno K, Gilstrap L. *Williams Obstetrics.* 19th ed. Norwalk, CT: Appleton & Lange, 1993.

DeCherney AH, Pernoll ML. *Current Obstetric & Gynecologic Diagnosis & Treatment.* 7th ed. Norwalk, CT: Appleton & Lange, 1994.

Eddy DM. *Common Screening Tests.* Philadelphia: American College of Physicians, 1991.

Eschenbach DA. History and review of bacterial vaginosis. *Am J Obstet Gynecol.* 1993;169:441–445.

Felig P, et al. *Endocrinology and Metabolism.* 2nd ed. New York: McGraw-Hill, 1987.

Fishbach F. *A Manual of Laboratory & Diagnostic Tests.* 4th ed. Philadelphia: JB Lippincott, 1992.

Gomel V, Munro MG, Rowe TC. *Gynecology: A practical approach.* Baltimore, MD: Williams & Wilkins, 1990.

Gray M. *Genitourinary Disorders.* St. Louis, MO: CV Mosby, 1992.

Haagensen C. *Diseases of the Breast.* 3rd ed. Philadelphia: WB Saunders, 1986.

Harris JR, et al. *Breast Diseases.* Philadelphia: JB Lippincott, 1991.

Hatcher RA, Stewart F, Trussell J. *Contraceptive Technology: 1990–1992.* 15th ed. New York: Irvington, 1992.

Houle A, Pickard CG, Ouimette R, Lohr J, Greenberg R. *Patient Guidelines for Nurse Practitioners.* 4th ed. Philadelphia: JB Lippincott, 1995.

Iams JD, Casal D, McGregor JA. Fetal fibronectin improves the accuracy of diagnosis of preterm labor. *Am J Obstet Gynecol.* 1995;173(1):141–145.

Institute of Medicine. *Prenatal Care: Reaching Mothers, Reaching Infants.* Washington, DC: National Academy Press, 1988.

Institute of Medicine. *Nutrition During Pregnancy: Summary.* Washington, DC: National Academy Press, 1990.

Joint American College of Obstetrics & Gynecology. *Guidelines for Labor and Delivery.* Washington, DC: Author, 1990.

Karch AM. *Lippincott's Nursing Drug Guide.* Philadelphia: JB Lippincott, 1996.

Keppel KG, Taffel SM. Pregnancy-related weight gain and retention: Implications of the 1990 Institute of Medicine Guidelines. *Am J Public Health.* 1993;83:1100–1103.

Lemke DP, Pattison J, Marshall LA, Cowley DS, eds. *Primary Care of Women.* Norwalk, CT: Appleton & Lange, 1995.

Lichtman R. Perimenopausal hormone replacement therapy: Review of the literature. *J Nurse Midwifery.* 1991;36:30–48.

Lichtman R, Papera S. *Gynecology Well Woman Care.* Norwalk, CT: Appleton & Lange, 1990.

Long P. Rethinking iron supplementation during pregnancy. *J Nurse Midwifery.* 1995;40(1):36–40.

Lossick JG, Kent HL. Trichomoniasis: Trends in diagnosis and management. *Am J Obstet Gynecol.* 1991;165:1217–1222.

Malasanos L, Barkauskas V, Stoltenberg-Allen K. *Health Assessment.* 4th ed. St. Louis, MO: CV Mosby, 1990.

Mays M. Tuberculosis: A comprehensive review for the certified nurse-midwife. *J Nurse Midwifery.* 1993;38(3):132–139.

McDonough J, ed. *Stedman's Concise Medical Dictionary.* 2nd ed. Baltimore, MD: Williams & Wilkins, 1993.

Medical Economics. *The PDR Family Guide to Nutrition and Health.* Montvale, NJ: Author, 1995.

Murphy P, Jones E. Use of oral metronidazole in pregnancy. *J Nurse Midwifery.* 1994;3(4):214–220.

Sibai BM. Definitive therapy of pregnancy-induced hypertension. *Contemporary OB/GYN.* May 1988:51–66.

Sitruk-Ware R, Bardin CW. *Contraception: Newer Pharmacological Agents, Devices, and Delivery Systems.* New York: Marcel Dekker, 1992.

Skidmore-Roth L. *Mosby's 1995 Nursing Drug Reference.* St. Louis, MO: CV Mosby, 1995.

Speroff L, Darney PD. *A Clinical Guide for Contraception.* Baltimore, MD: Williams & Wilkins, 1992.

Star W, Shannon M, Sammons L, Lommel L, Gutierrez Y. *Ambulatory Obstetrics: Protocols for Nurse Practitioners/Nurse Midwives.* 2nd ed. San Francisco, CA: School of Nursing, University of California Press, 1990.

Stine GJ. *The Biology of Sexually Transmitted Diseases.* Dubuque, IA: WC Brown, 1992.

Sweet RL, Gibbs RS. *Infectious Diseases of the Female Genital Tract.* 2nd ed. Baltimore, MD: Williams & Wilkins, 1990.

Tierney LM Jr, McPhee SJ, Papadakis MA, Schroeder SA, eds. *Current Medical Diagnosis & Treatment.* Norwalk, CT: Appleton & Lange, 1993.

U.S. Department of Health and Human Services, Public Health Service. *Caring for Our Future: The Content of Prenatal Care.* Washington, DC: Author, 1989.

U.S. Department of Health and Human Services, Public Health Service. *1989 Sexually Transmitted Diseases Treatment Guidelines.* Atlanta, GA: Centers for Disease Control, 1989.

U.S. Department of Health and Human Services, Public Health Service. *Healthy People 2000: National Health Promotion and Disease Prevention Objectives* (DHHS Pub. No. 91-50212). Washington, DC: United States Government Office, 1991.

Varney H. *Nurse-Midwifery.* Boston, MA: Blackwell Scientific, 1986.

Weil EK, Murphy JL, Burke J, eds. *Nurse Practitioners Prescribing Reference.* New York: Prescribing Reference Inc, 1995.

Wistreich GA. *The Sexually Transmitted Diseases: A Current Approach.* Dubuque, IA: WC Brown, 1992.

Women's Health Collective. *The All New Our Bodies, Ourselves.* New York: Simon & Schuster, 1984.

Wright VC, Lickrish GM, eds. *Basic and Advanced Colposcopy.* Houston, TX: Biomedical Communications, 1989.

APPENDIX I

Topical Agents

Drug	Brand Name	Recommended Dosage	Considerations
Adrenocorticoids			
Medrol		Apply small amount and gently rub into skin.	Relieves redness, swelling, and itching caused by hemorrhoid discomfort, insect bites, poison ivy, oak, sumac, soaps, cosmetics, and jewelry.
Anesthetics			
	Americaine spray; Dibucaine ointment; Nupercainal ointment	Use only enough to cover irritation.	Relieves pain and itch of sunburn, insect bites, scratches, hemorrhoids, and other minor skin irritations.
Lidocaine hydrochloride	Lidocaine	Viscous solution: 1%, 2% (1–2 mg/ml). Dose varies with area to be anesthetized. Use lowest dose possible to achieve desired results.	Relieves burning, stinging, tenderness, and tissue irritations.
Antibiotics			
Mupirocin	Bactroban	Apply small amount to affected area three times a day. Can be covered with gauze dressing.	Use to treat impetigo caused by *S. aureus*, streptococci, and *S. pyogens*. Monitor for signs of superinfection; reevaluate if no response in 3–5 d.
	Neosporin	Apply small amount every 3–4 hr for 7–10 d.	Prevents infection due to minor cuts, scrapes, and burns.
Antifungals			
Clotrimazole	Lotrimin; Mycelex	Gently massage into affected area twice a day.	Cleanse area before applying; use for up to 4 wk. Discontinue if irritation occurs or condition worsens.

Econazole nitrate	Spectazole	Apply locally twice a day.	Use for athlete's foot; change socks and shoes at least once a day. Cleanse area before applying; treat for 2–4 wk. Discontinue if irritation or burning occurs or condition worsens.
Gentian violet		Apply locally twice a day.	May stain skin and clothes; DO NOT apply to active lesions.
Naftifine HCl	Naftin	Gently massage into affected area twice a day.	Avoid occlusive dressings; wash hands thoroughly after application. DO NOT use longer than 4 wk.
Oxiconazole	Oxistat	Apply twice every day.	May need for up to 1 mo.
Terbinafine	Lamisil	Apply to area twice a day until clinical signs improve; 1–4 wk.	DO NOT use occlusive dressings; report local irritations. Discontinue if local irritation occurs.
Tolnaftate	Tinactin; Genaspor; Ting; Aftate	Apply small amount twice a day for 2–3 wk; 4–6 wk may be necessary if skin is thick.	Cleanse skin with soap and water before application; dry thoroughly. Wear loose, well-fitted shoes; change socks at least four times a day.
Antipsoriatics			
Ammoniated mercury	Emersal	Apply twice every day.	Protect from light; potential sensitizer provoking severe allergic reactions.
Anthralin	Anthra-Derm; Lasan; Dritho-Creme	Apply every day only to psoriatic lesions.	May stain fabrics, skin, hair, nails; use protective dressing.
Antiseborrheics			
Selenium sulfide	Selsun Blue; Exsel	Massage 5–10 ml into scalp; allow to sit 2–3 min, then rinse.	Remove jewelry before use; may damage. Discontinue if irritation occurs.

(*continued*)

Drug	Brand Name	Recommended Dosage	Considerations
Emollients			
Boric acid ointment	Borofax	Apply as needed.	Relieves burns, itching, irritation.
Dexpanthenol	Panthoderm	Apply twice every day.	Relieves itching and aids in healing mild skin irritations.
Glycerin		Combined with other ingredients—rose water.	Moisturizing effect.
Lanolin		Ointment based, apply generously.	Allergy to sheep or sheep products—use caution; base for many ointments.
Eucerin		Apply as needed.	Relieves dry skin and pruritus.
Vitamin A acid, tretinoin derivative	Retin-A	Initially apply to cleansed and completely dry skin once daily at bedtime. Adjust strength or frequency as tolerated and needed.	Use for acne vulgaris.
Vitamins A and D		Apply locally with gentle massage twice to four times a day.	Relieves minor burns, chafing, skin irritations. Consult physician if no improvement within 7 d.
Zinc oxide		Apply as needed.	Relieves burns, abrasions, diaper rash.
Keratolytics			
Benzoyl peroxide	Persa-Gel; Benzagel 14% gel	Apply to cleansed area 1–2 times daily. Avoid mouth and mucous membranes.	Relief of acne vulgaris.
	Desquam	Massage into cleansed area 1–2 times daily. Avoid mouth, eyes, and mucous membranes.	Relief of mild to moderate acne.
Podofilox	Condylox	Apply every 12 hr for 3 consecutive days.	Allow area to dry before usage. Dispose of used applicator; may cause burning and discomfort.

Lotions/Solutions

Burow's solution aluminum acetate	Bluboro Powder Boropak Powder; Domeboro Powder; Pedi-Boro Soak Paks	Dissolve one packet in a pint of water, apply four times a day for 30 min.	Astringent wet dressing for relief of inflammatory conditions, insect bites, athlete's foot, bruise, etc; do not use occlusive dressing.
Calamine lotion	Calamox; Resinol; Calamatum	Apply to affected area three to four times a day.	Relieves itching, pain of poison ivy, sumac, and oak; insect bites; and other minor skin irritations.
Hammamelis water	Witch Hazel; Tucks; A.E.R.	Apply locally up to six times a day.	Relieves itching and irritation of vaginal infection, hemorrhoids, postepisiotomy discomfort, post-hemorrhoidectomy.

Pediculicides/Scabicides

Lindane	Kwell; Scabene; G-Well	Apply thin layer to entire body and leave 8–12 hr; then wash thoroughly. Shampoo 1–2 oz into hair and leave 4 min.	For extreme use only. Single application usually sufficient. Reapply after 7 d if sign of live lice. Ensure all contacts are treated. Disease is readily communicated. Teach hygiene and prevention.
Crotamiton	Eurax	Thoroughly massage onto entire body; repeat in 24 hr. Take cleansing bath or shower 48 hr after application.	For external use only. Shake well before using. Change bed linens and clothing the next day. Contaminated clothes can be dry cleaned or washed on hot cycle.
Permethrin	Nix, Elimite	Thoroughly massage into skin (30 g/adult); wash off after 8–14 hr. Shampoo into freshly washed, rinsed, and towel-dried hair. Leave on 10 min and rinse.	For external use only. Single application is usually curative. Notify health care provider if rash and/or itching worsens.

Index

References followed by "t" denote tables

A

abortion, spontaneous, 85–86, 117–118
abruptio placenta, 67–68, 68t
acetaminophen, 279, 312
　with codeine, 313
acne, 214
acquired hemolytic anemia, 75–76
Actifed, 258
acyclovir, 155, 259
Adrenalin, 272
adrenal insufficiency, 110
adrenocorticoids, 322t
Advil, 284
AER, 325t
Aftate, 323t
albuterol, 303
alendronate, 282
alopecia, during pregnancy, 226
aluminum acetate, 325t
amenorrhea
　clinical features, 69–70
　definition of, 69
　etiology of, 69
　laboratory studies, 69–70
　management of, 70–71
　oral contraceptive use and, 25
　pharmacologic treatment, 70–71
Americaine spray, 322t
amniocentesis, 135
amniotomy, 35
amoxicillin, 259
Amoxil, 259
ampicillin, 260
anemia
　acquired hemolytic, 75–76
　clinical features, 72
　criteria for physician consultation, 74
　definition of, 72
　etiology of, 72
　iron deficiency, 77–78
　management of, 72–74
　megaloblastic, 79
　pernicious, 80
　sickle cell, 81
anesthetics, 322t
antepartum visits, considerations for
　initial visit, 26–27
　return visit, 28–29
Anthra-Derm, 323t
anthralin, 323t
antibacterial agents. *See specific drug*
antibiotics. *See specific drug*
antifungals, 323t
antipsoriatics, 323t
antiseborrheics, 323t
Anxanil, 314
Apo-Prednisone, 297
appendicitis, 118
arteriolar vasospasm, 144
aspirin, 261, 279
Atarax, 314
athlete's foot, 214–215
atrophic vaginitis, 250
autosomal disorders, 133
azithromycin, 315
AZT, 262

B

backache, 82
back pain. *See* low back pain; upper back pain
bacterial vaginosis, 83–84
Bactroban, 322t
basal body temperature family planning method, 18–19
Bayer, 261
Bellergal-S, 263
Benadryl, 264
Benzagel, 324t
benzoyl peroxide, 324t
betamethasone diproprionate, 264
Bicillin Long-Acting, 265
Bishop's score, 199t
bleeding during pregnancy
　over 20 weeks' gestation, 89–90
　under 20 weeks' gestation, 85–88
blood pressure screening, 5t
blood sugar testing, 45
blood type testing, 41
bloody show, 89
Bluboro Powder, 325t
boric acid ointment, 324t
Borofax, 324t
Boropak Powder, 325t
breakthrough bleeding, 24

breastfeeding, chlamydia treatment during, 98
breasts
  physical examination of, 4
  screening recommendations, 5t
breech presentation, 91
Burow's solution, 325t
butalbital, 279
butoconazole nitrate, 278
butorphanol tartrate, 309

C

caffeine, 279
Calamatum, 325t
calamine lotion, 325t
Calamox, 325t
calcium carbonate, 312
carboprost tromethamine, 283
carbuncles, 217
cardiovascular assessment, 92–93
cardiovascular disease, 177
care during pregnancy. *See* pregnancy care
CBC with differential, 41
ceftriaxone sodium, 306
Celestone Soluspan, 264
cephalexin, 286
cervical abnormalities, 89, 94–95
cervical cancer, 86, 187
cervical cap, 8–9
cervical culture, 46
cervical mucous family planning method, 19
cervical polyps, 86
cervicitis, 94, 250–251
cervix, normal hyperemia of, 86
chickenpox. *See* varicella zoster
chlamydia
  clinical features, 96–97
  culture testing, 44–45
  etiology of, 96
  incidence of, 96
  laboratory testing, 98
  management of, 97–98
  pharmacologic treatment, 99
chloasma, during pregnancy, 226
chloraxine, 323t
cholestatic jaundice, 210
cholestyramine, 266
chorionic villi sampling, 135
chromagen, 266
chromosomal aberrations, 133–134
cirrhosis, 110
Cleocin/Cleocin Vaginal, 267
Climara, 268
clindamycin hydrochloride, 267
clotrimazole, 322t
clotting time testing, 46
Colace, 268

colds, 99
colonoscopy screening, 6t
condom, 9–10
condylomata acuminata, 159–160
Condylox, 324t
conjunctivitis, chronic, 96
constipation, 50t-51t
contact dermatitis, 215
contraception
  discussion with patient, 7
  method desired, factors that affect, 7–8
contraceptive methods
  cervical cap, 8–9
  condom, 9–10
  Depo-Provera, 10–11, 270
  diaphragm, 11–14
  intrauterine device, 14–18
  natural family planning, 18–20
  Norplant, 20–21, 292
  oral contraceptives. *See* oral contraceptives
  spermicides, 25
coughs, 100–101
coxsackie B enterovirus, 227
crabs. *See* pediculosis pubis
crotamiton, 325t
culture testing
  chlamydia, 44–45
  gonorrhea, 44
  herpes simplex, 45
  urine, 43
cystitis, 244–245

D

Darvocet-N 100, 269
delivery, of baby. *See* labor
Delta-Cortef, 296
Deltasone, 297
Demerol, 269
dependent edema, 50t-51t
Depo-Provera, 10–11, 270
dermatitis
  contact, 215
  seborrheic, 220
Desquam, 324t
dexpanthenol, 324t
diabetes mellitus
  clinical features, 102–103
  complications of, 106
  definition of, 102
  diagnosis, 103–104
  etiology of, 102
  insulin, 102
  laboratory testing, 104–105
  management of, 104–106
  signs and symptoms of, 104
diaphragm
  advantages and disadvantages, 11
  contraindications, 12

definition of, 11
effectiveness of, 11
fitting, 13
management of, 12–14
diarrhea, 107–108
Dibucaine ointment, 322t
Diflucan, 270
dinoprostone, 303
diphenhydramine hydrochloride, 264
Dipstix urine test, 43–44
discharge, vaginal. *See* vaginal discharge
discomforts, of pregnancy
  constipation, 50t–51t
  dependent edema, 51t–52t
  dyspareunia, 52t
  fatigue, 52t–53t
  gas, 53t
  headache, 53t–54t
  heartburn, 54t–55t
  hemorrhoids, 55t–56t
  insomnia, 56t–57t
  leg cramps, 57t
  leukorrhea, 58t
  low back pain, 49t
  nausea, 58t–59t
  nocturia, 60t
  round ligament pain, 60t–61t
  shortness of breath, 61t
  supine hypotensive syndrome, 62t
  tingling and numbness of fingers, 62t
  upper back pain, 50t
  varicosities, 63t
docusate, 268, 307
Domeboro Powder, 325t
Down syndrome, incidence of, 134
doxycycline, 271
doxylamine succinate, 313
Dritho-Creme, 323t
drugs. *See specific drug*
dysfunctional uterine bleeding, 109–111
dysmenorrhea
  clinical features, 112–114
  etiology of, 112
  incidence of, 112
  management of, 114–116
dyspareunia, 52t

E

econazole nitrate, 323t
Ecotrin, 261
ectopic pregnancy, 117–118
eczema, 215–216
EDC. *See* estimated date of confinement
edema, 50t–51t, 119–120
E.E.S., 273
Elimite, 325t
Emersal, 323t
Emetrol, 271
emollients, 324t

Empirin, 261
E-mycin, 273
endometrial biopsy, 121–122
endometriosis
  clinical features, 94, 113
  puerperal infection and, differential diagnosis, 212–213
  treatment of, 115
endometritis
  clinical features of, 123–124
  definition of, 123
  etiology of, 123
  management of, 124–125
  pharmacologic treatment of, 124–125
endosalpinigitis, 137
Engerix-B, 283
Entex/Entex LA, 272
epinephrine, 272
erythromycin ethylsuccinate, 273
esterified estrogens, 276
estimated date of confinement, 126–127
Estrace, 274
Estraderm transdermal patch, 275
estradiol, 268, 274–275
Estratest/Estratest H.S., 276
estrogen, 142, 276, 298
estropipate, 294
ethambutol, 277
eucerin, 324t
Eurax, 325t
Excedrin IB, 284
Exsel, 323t

F

famciclovir sodium, 277
family planning, natural. *See* natural family planning
Famvir, 277
fatigue, 52t–53t
Femstat, 278
Feosol, 278
Fer-iron, 278
Ferospace, 278
ferrous sulfate, 278
fetal fibronectin, 208
fetus. *See also* neonate
  diabetes mellitus effects, 102, 106
  genetic screening. *See* genetic screening
  gonorrhea effects, 138–139
  heart tones, 128–129
  hepatitis effects, 149–150
  herpes simplex infection effects, 156
  intrauterine growth retardation, 166–167
  non-stress test, 186
  polyhydramnios effects, 196
  rubella effects, 223
  in utero movement of, 130–131
fFN. *See* fetal fibronectin

fibroids, uterine, 113–114
fifth disease, 227
fingers, tingling and numbness of, 62t
Fioricet, 279
Fiorinal, 279
Flagyl, 280
Fleet Enema, 280
Floxin, 281
flu, 99
fluconazole, 270
fluorescent treponema antibody test, 233–234
flu vaccinations, 248
folic acid, 281
folliculitis, 216–217
foreign objects, in vagina, 250
Fosamax, 282
FTA test. *See* fluorescent treponema antibody test
furuncles, 217

G

galactorrhea, 132
Gamastan, 285
Gammar, 285
Genaspor, 323t
genetic screening
   autosomal dominant disorders, 133
   autosomal recessive disorders, 133
   chromosomal aberrations, 133–134
   patient groups at high risk, 134–135
   sex-linked disorders, 133
genital warts. *See* condylomata acuminata
gentian violet, 323t
glucose metabolism, 102
glucose tolerance test, 104–105
glycerin, 324t
   suppositories, 282
gonorrhea
   course of, 137
   culture testing, 44
   definition of, 137
   differential diagnosis, 139
   etiology of, 137
   fetal effects, 138–139
   management of, 139
   pelvic inflammatory disease, 138
   pregnancy effects, 138
   signs and symptoms of, 137–138
   treatment, 139–140
G6PD deficiencies. *See* acquired hemolytic anemia
grand multiparity, 141
GTT. *See* glucose tolerance test
G-Well, 325t
gynecologic care. *See also specific disease*
   history taking, 3
   physical examination, 3–4
   screening tests, 4, 5t-6t

H

hammamelis water, 325t
headache, 53t–54t, 142–143
heartburn, 54t–55t
heart tones, fetal, 128–129
HELLP syndrome, 144–145
Hemabate, 283
hemoccult nonfasting cholesterol screening recommendations, 6t
hemorrhage, postpartum. *See* postpartum hemorrhage
hemorrhoids, 55t–56t, 146
heparin lock, 35
hepatitis
   clinical features of, 148–149
   definition of, 147
   etiology of, 147
   fetal and neonatal considerations, 149–150
   management of, 150–151
   maternal considerations, 149
   pruritis during pregnancy and, differential diagnosis, 210
   types of, 147, 148t
   vaccinations, 248, 283
Heptovax, 283
herpes simplex virus
   clinical features, 152–154
   culture testing, 45
   definition of, 152
   diagnosis of, 153–154
   etiology of, 152
   fetal and neonatal considerations, 156
   management of, 154–156
   pharmacologic treatment, 155
   during pregnancy, 229t
   primary *vs.* recurrent, signs and symptoms of, 153t
high blood pressure, during pregnancy. *See* hypertension during pregnancy
hirsutism, 226
history taking, 3. *See also specific disease*
HIV. *See* human immunodeficiency viral disease
hives, 217–218
hormone replacement therapy, 179–180
HPV. *See* human papilloma virus
HRT. *See* hormone replacement therapy
HSV. *See* herpes simplex virus
human immunodeficiency viral disease
   description of, 157–158
   zidovudine treatment, 262
human papilloma virus, 94, 159–160, 187
hydatidiform mole, 161–162
hydroxychloroquine, 284
hydroxyzine hydrochloride, 314
hyperpigmentation, 226
hypertension during pregnancy
   clinical features, 163

definition of, 163
  management of, 164–165
hyperthyroidism, 238
hypothyroidism, 238

I

Ibuprin, 284
ibuprofen, 284
immune globulin, 285
impetigo, 218–219, 229t
implantation bleeding, 85
influenza pneumonia, 193–194
influenza vaccinations. *See* flu vaccinations
INH, 286
insomnia, 56t–57t
insulin, 102. *See also* diabetes mellitus
intrauterine device
  advantages and disadvantages, 14
  contraindications, 14–15
  definition of, 14
  effectiveness of, 14
  insertion procedure, 16
  management of, 15–16
  pregnancy and, 18
  removal of, 17–18
  side effects and complications, 17
intrauterine fetal growth retardation, 166–167
iron, 308
iron deficiency anemia, 77–78
isoimmunization
  clinical features, 168–169
  definition of, 168
  incidence of, 168
  management of, 169–170
  patient education, 170
isoniazid, 286
IUD. *See* intrauterine device
IUFGR. *See* intrauterine fetal growth retardation

K

Keflex, 286
keratolytics, 324t
ketoconazole, 291
Kwell, 325t

L

labor. *See also* pregnancy
  consultation and/or collaborative management, 39–40
  fetal heart tone monitoring, 128–129
  medication, 36
  ongoing management of, 34–38
  onset of, methods to determine, 33–34
  oxytocin induction or augmentation, 40–41
  physician referral, 39–40
  postmaturity, 198–199
  postpartum care. *See* postpartum care
  premature rupture of membranes. *See* membranes, premature rupture of
  prematurity, 207–209
  stages of, 34–36
laboratory studies, for pregnancy care, 27–28, 41–46
Lamisil, 323t
lanolin, 324t
Lasan, 323t
leg cramps, 57t
leukorrhea, 58t
levonorgestrel, 292
Lidocaine, 322t
lindane, 325t
liver disease, 210
Lotrimin, 322t
low back pain, 49t
lupus, 171–172
lymphogranuloma venereum, 96

M

Macrobid, 287
Macrodantin, 287
magnesium hydroxide, 290
magnesium sulfate, 288
mammography, 5t, 173
mastitis, 174–175
Medrol, 322t
medroxyprogesterone acetate, 270, 304
megaloblastic anemia, 79
membranes, premature rupture of
  definition of, 204
  etiology of, 204
  management of, 204–206
menopause
  clinical features, 176–177
  definition of, 176
  etiology of, 176
  management of, 177–180
  pharmacologic treatment, 178–180
menstrual disorders. *See* amenorrhea; dysmenorrhea
meperidine, 269
Meruvax II, 307
Metamucil, 288
Methergine, 289
methylergonovine maleate, 289
methyltestosterone, 276
MetroGel-Vaginal, 289
metronidazole, 280, 289
miconazole, 291
Micronor, 290
Midol IB, 284
migraine, 142–143

Milk of Magnesia, 290
molluscum contagiosum, 219
moniliasis, 219–220
Monistat 3, 291
Monistat 7, 291
Motrin, 284
multiple pregnancy, 184–185
mupirocin, 322t
Myambutol, 277
Mycelex, 322t
Mycostatin, 293

N

naftifine hydrochloride, 323t
Naftin, 323t
natural family planning
  advantages and disadvantages, 18
  contraindications, 18
  definition of, 18
  effectiveness of, 18
  methods of, 18–20
nausea, 58t–59t
Neisseria gonorrhoeae. See gonorrhea
neonate. *See also* fetus
  hepatitis effects, 150
  herpes simplex infection effects, 156
Neosporin, 322t
nitrofurantoin, 287
Nix, 325t
Nizoral, 291
nocturia, 60t
nonoxynol 9, 292
non-stress test, 186
norethindrone, 290
Norplant
  advantages and disadvantages, 20
  complications, 21
  contraindications, 20
  definition of, 20
  description of, 292
  effectiveness of, 20
  management of, 21
Novoprednisolone, 296
Nucofed, 293
Nupercainal ointment, 322t
Nuprin, 284
nutrition requirements during pregnancy, 31–32
nystatin, 293

O

ofloxacin, 281
Ogen tablets/vaginal cream, 294
omnipen, 260
oral contraceptives
  advantages and disadvantages, 21–22
  contraindications, 22
  definition of, 21
  effectiveness of, 21
  follow-up, 24–25
  initiation of, 22–23
  instructions to patient, 23–24
  management of, 22–25
osteoporosis, 177
ovarian cyst, 118
ovulation kits, for family planning, 20
oxiconazole, 323t
Oxistat, 323t
oxytocin, 40–41, 295

P

Pamprin-IB, 284
Panasol, 297
Panthoderm, 324t
Papanicolaou (Pap) smear
  classification system, 187t
  definition of, 187
  management of, 188
  during pregnancy, 44
  screening recommendations, 5t
papular eruptions, during pregnancy, 228t
parasites testing, 46
Pedi-Boro Soak Paks, 325t
pediculicides, 325t
pediculosis pubis, 189–190
pelvic examination, 4
pelvic inflammatory disease
  clinical features, 113
  ectopic pregnancy and, differential diagnosis, 118
  treatment of, 115
penicillin G benzathine, 265
perimenopause
  clinical features, 176–177
  definition of, 176
  etiology of, 176
  management of, 177–180
  pharmacologic treatment, 178–180
permethrin, 325t
pernicious anemia, 80
Persa-Gel, 324t
Phenergan/Phenergan VC, 294
Phenergan suppository, 302
physical examination, 3–4. *See also specific disease*
physician referral during labor, situations that warrant, 39–40
"pill." *See* oral contraceptives
Pitocin, 295
placenta previa, 89, 191–192
Plaquenil, 284
platelet count, during pregnancy, 46
pneumonia
  clinical features, 193–194
  definition of, 193
  etiology of, 193

influenza, 193
  management of, 194–195
  Streptococcus, 194
  varicella-zoster, 194
podofilox, 324t
polyhydramnios, 196–197
polyps
  cervical, 86
  clinical features of, 94
postmaturity, 198–199
postpartum care
  in hospital, 36–38
  in office, 38
postpartum hemorrhage
  fourth stage, 200–202
  late, 202–203
  third stage, 200
prednisolone, 296
prednisone, 297
preeclampsia
  edema and, differential diagnosis, 119
  signs and symptoms of, 163
pregnancy. *See also* labor
  bleeding during. *See* bleeding during pregnancy
  care during. *See* pregnancy care
  common discomforts during. *See* discomforts, of pregnancy
  ectopic, 117–118
  hypertension. *See* hypertension during pregnancy
  intrauterine device use and, 18
  iron deficiency anemia. *See* iron deficiency anemia
  laboratory studies, 41–46
  multiple, 184–185
  nutritional requirements, 31–32
  skin conditions. *See* skin conditions, during pregnancy
  weight gain, 31–33
pregnancy care
  collaborative care and referral, 29–31
  initial antepartum visit, 26–27
  objectives of, 26
  philosophy, 25–26
  return antepartum visit, 28–29
Prelone, 296
Premarin vaginal cream, 298
prematurity, 207–209
Premphase, 299
Prempro, 300
prenatal laboratory studies, 41–46
Preparation H, 300
Prepidil gel, 303
Principen, 260
probenecid, 301
Proctofoam-HC, 301
progesterone, 142
  in oil, 302
promethazine hydrochloride, 302

propoxyphene napsylate with acetaminophen, 269
Prostin E2, 303
prothrombin time testing, 46
Proventil inhaler, 303
Provera, 304
pruritus, in pregnancy, 210–211, 228t
pseudoephedrine hydrochloride, 258, 309
psyllium, 288
puerperal infection, 212–213
pyelonephritis, 213, 244
Pyrazinamide, 305

Q
Questran Light, 266
quickening, 130

R
ranitidine, 314
rapid plasma reagin (RPR) test, 233
rashes. *See also* skin conditions, during pregnancy
  acne, 214
  athlete's foot, 214–215
  carbuncles, 217
  contact dermatitis, 215
  eczema, 215–216
  folliculitis, 216–217
  furuncles, 217
  hives, 217–218
  impetigo, 218–219
  molluscum contagiosum, 219
  moniliasis, 219–220
  seborrheic dermatitis, 220
Resinol, 325t
Retin-A, 324t
Retrovir, 262
Rh factor testing, 41
Rho(D) immune globulin human, 305
RhoGAM, 169–170, 192, 305
rhythm method, 20
Rifadin, 306
rifampin, 306
Rocephin, 306
round ligament pain, 60t–61t, 221
rubella
  clinical features, 222–223
  managment of, 222–223
  testing, 42
  vaccinations, 248, 307

S
SAB. *See* spontaneous abortion
Scabene, 325t
scabicides, 325t
scabies, 210, 224–225

screening tests
  evaluation of, 4
  genetic. *See* genetic screening
  mammography. *See* mammography
  Papanicolaou (Pap) smear. *See* Papanicolaou (Pap) smear
  types of, 5t–6t
seborrheic dermatitis, 220
selenium sulfide, 323t
Selsun Blue, 323t
Semicid, 292
Senokot, 307
serology testing, 41
serum alpha-fetoprotein testing, 42–43, 135
serum pregnancy testing, 46
sex-linked disorders, 133
sexually transmitted diseases
  chlamydia. *See* chlamydia
  condylomata acuminata, 159–160
  gonorrhea. *See* gonorrhea
  herpes simplex virus. *See* herpes simplex virus
  human immunodeficiency viral disease, 157–158
  pediculosis pubis, 189–190
  syphilis. *See* syphilis
  Trichomonas vaginitis, 240–241
shortness of breath, during pregnancy, 61t
sickle cell anemia, 81
sickle cell screen, 42
sigmoidoscopy screening, 6t
skin conditions, during pregnancy. *See also* rashes
  chloasma, 226
  herpes gestations, 229t
  hirsutism/alopecia, 226
  hyperpigmentation, 226
  impetigo herpetiformis, 229t
  papular eruptions, 228t
  pruritic urticarial papules, 228t
  pruritus gravidarum, 228t
  striae, 226
  vascular distention, 226–227
skin disease, 210
"slapped face" syndrome. *See* fifth disease
Slow Fe, 308
sodium biphosphate, 280
sodium intake, 119
sore throat, 231
Spectazole, 323t
spectinomycin, 308
spermicides, 25. *See also* nonoxynol 9
spontaneous abortion, 85–86, 117–118
Stadol, 309
STDs. *See* sexually transmitted diseases
streptococcus pneumonia, 194

striae, during pregnancy, 226
Sudafed, 309
supine hypotensive syndrome, 62t
syphilis
  acquired, 232–233
  clinical features, 232–233
  congenital, 233
  definition of, 232
  etiology of, 232
  laboratory testing, 233–234
  management of, 234–235
  treatment of, 234–235
systemic lupus erythematosus. *See* lupus
systolic murmur, 92

T

Terazol, 310
terbinafine, 323t
terbutaline, 310
terconazole, 310
tetracycline, 311
thrombophlebitis, 213, 236–237
thyroid disease, 238–239
thyroid screen testing, 45
Tigan, 311
Tinactin, 323t
tinea pedis. *See* athlete's foot
Ting, 323t
tingling and numbness of fingers, during pregnancy, 62t
tolnaftate, 323t
topical agents. *See specific drug*
toxoplasmosis, 27
Treponema pallidum. *See* syphilis
tretinoin, 324t
Trichomonas vaginitis, 240–241
trimethobenzamide hydrochloride, 311
trimox, 259
triprolidine hydrochloride, 258
Trobicin, 308
tuberculosis, 242–243
Tucks, 325t
Tums, 312
Tylenol, 312
Tylenol 3, 313

U

ultrasonography, 28
Unisom, 313
upper back pain, 50t
upper respiratory infection, 99
urethritis, 244
urinalysis testing, 43
urinary tract infection
  clinical features, 244–245
  definitions, 244

differential diagnosis, 245
etiology of, 244
management of, 245–246
puerperal infection and, differential diagnosis, 213
self-help measures, 247
treatment of, 246
urine culture and sensitivity testing, 43
urogenital atrophy, 176–177
urticaria. *See* hives
uterine fibroids, 113–114
uterine prolapse
clinical features, 113
treatment of, 116
uterine rupture, 89

V

vaccinations, 248
vaginal discharge
clinical features, 251–253
etiology of, 249–251
incidence of, 249
infectious, 251. *See also specific disease*
management of, 253–254
noninfectious, 249–250
physical examination, 252–253
treatment of, 254

vaginosis, bacterial, 83–84
varicella zoster
pneumonia, 194
during pregnancy, 227, 230
varicosities, 63t
vascular distention, 226–227
VDRL test, 41–42, 233
Vibramycin, 271
Vistaril, 314
vitamin A, 324t
vitamin D, 324t

W

warts, genital. *See* condylomata acuminata
weight gain during pregnancy, 31–33
wet mount, 46
Witch Hazel, 325t

Z

Zantac, 314
zidovudine, 262
zinc oxide, 324t
Zithromax, 315
Zovirax, 259

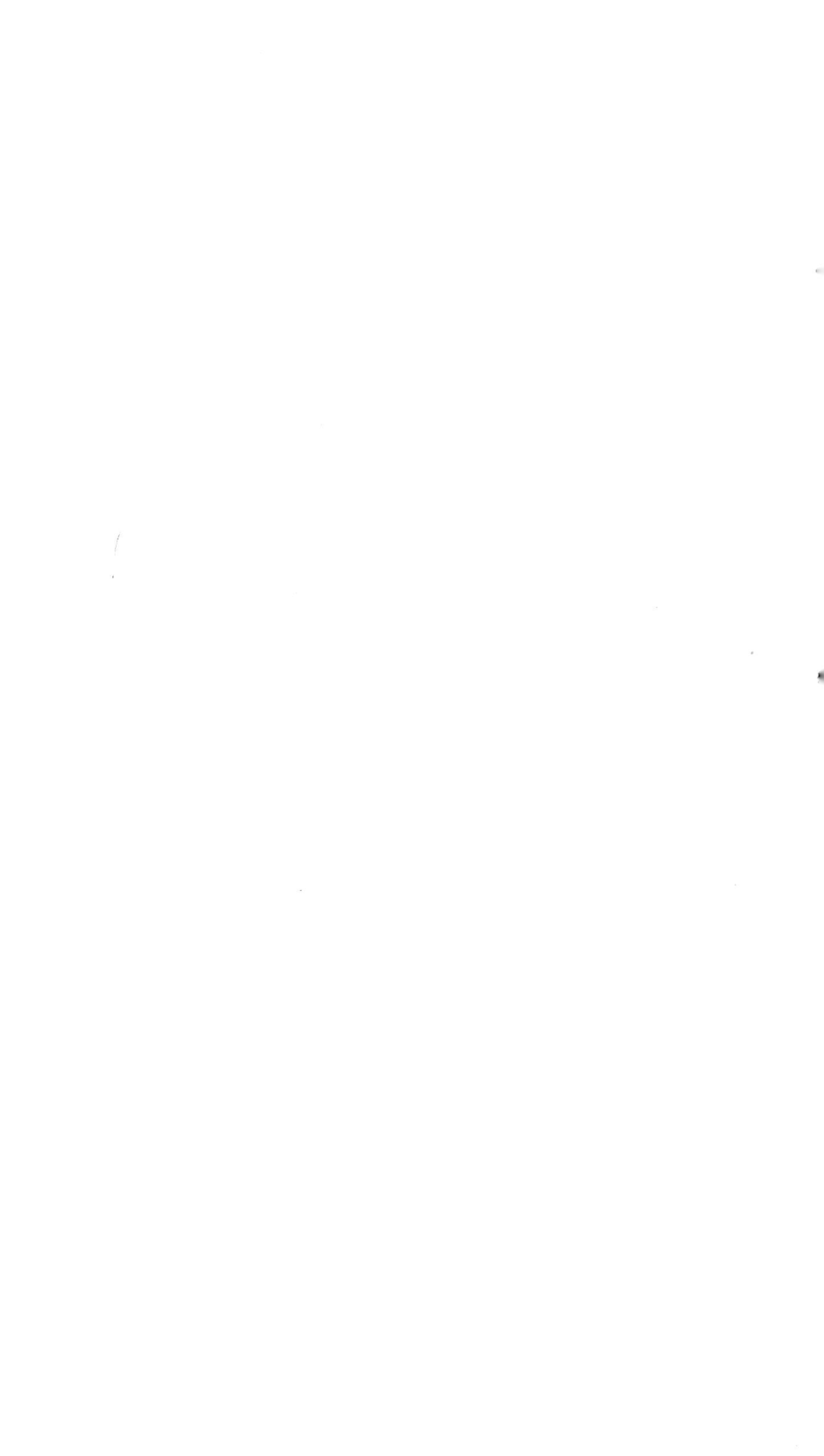